Dear Laura,

Autism is a lifelong journey.
Best wishes,
Linda A Ruth

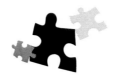

ONE IN
TEN THOUSAND

FOR THE LOVE OF LEE,
A MOTHER'S STORY.

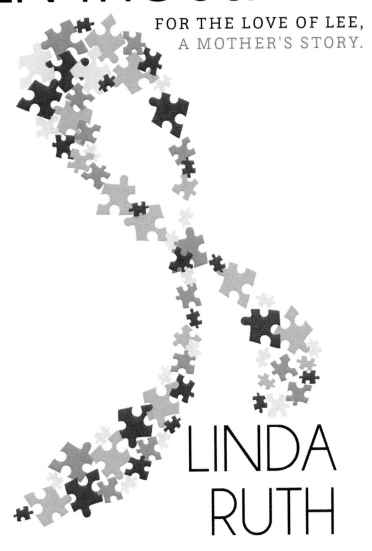

LINDA
RUTH

One in Ten Thousand
©2021 Linda Ruth

Print ISBN 978-1-66782-012-5
eBook ISBN 978-1-66782-013-2

This book details the life, trials, and challenges of Lee Ruth, as seen through the eyes of his mother, who is his advocate, champion, and caregiver. Lee struggled as a child when diagnosed as autistic in the 1970s. This book captures the struggles, adversity, perseverance, love, and hope that have been a hallmark of his journey to living a fulfilling life.

This book is dedicated to Zach, Ben, Abby, Brady, and Colin. You are my reasons for writing. Always believe in miracles.

CONTENTS

PREFACE

*"The journey of a thousand miles begins
with a single step."*

–Lao Tzu

A random call from my older brother changed my way of dealing with my son's autism, "Go for a run," he told me. *Go for a run? How could I possibly find a minute, let alone ten minutes, to run and for what purpose?* "It will help clear your mind," he said.

At the time, my mind was heavy with worry. My youngest son was eighteen months old; my oldest son was seven years old; and my middle son, Lee, who was almost five years old had been diagnosed with autism two years earlier. I cried often. I didn't want my children to see me struggling, so I retreated to my bedroom for a few minutes to take a deep breath and gather myself. The demands of early-childhood-intervention therapies, child-psychiatry appointments, and fear for Lee's future, on top of the typical day-to-day needs of raising three little boys, were taking a toll on me.

I always admired my older brother. He jogged regularly and was an outstanding athlete in high school. So, one day, I laced up an old pair of tennis shoes and ran one lap around our yard, about a quarter mile. I came back into the house panting, my legs feeling like rubber. I struggled to take a load of wash downstairs. I was exhausted, but surprisingly I felt good enough to try it the next day and then the next, always feeling a bit better when I finished. I noticed it really did help to clear my mind. I didn't feel as defeated. I realized jogging was actually helping me feel better in a subtle way.

Little-by-little, step-by-step, running the next day and then the next was the beginning of my twenty-five-year love of running. It reflects the way I have coped, all of these years, with my son's autism.

As a little girl growing up in middle-class suburbia, I was always a competitor. Not the type of competitor who had to win, but the type of competitor who put her nose to the grindstone and gutted it out. Like running, I was always willing to go the distance. Little did I know I was preparing for my life ahead as the mother of a child with special needs.

Through my fun-loving childhood and the influence of my father, with all the laughter and funny antics, I learned to see the light and humorous side of life's situations. My hard-working parents, first generation Americans of Polish immigrants, ingrained a faith and a genuine love of family that set the foundation in my quest in dealing with my problems in years to come, problems I never even knew existed at the time.

What is autism?

Navigating autism in the late 1970s and 1980s was not easy. Only a handful of specialists had even an inkling of what was going on. Lee's diagnosis came in 1976, a time in autism's history when many so-called experts still cruelly blamed mothers for causing this disability. The theory was that emotional trauma from cold and rejecting mothers triggered children to protect themselves by turning inward. Everyone now knows that the truth is quite the opposite: the undying love of mothers of autistic children is what kept the quest for answers alive since the earliest diagnosis of this puzzling disability, and it is what led to the understanding and acceptance of autism that exists today. I recognized early on that to help Lee, I was going to have to be the one to search for the answers.

This is the story of my undying love for Lee. It's about my refusal to accept Lee's diagnosis of autism, when one child in ten thousand, instead of today's one, in forty-four, is diagnosed. It's a story about refusing to submit to the status quo and fighting to ensure Lee's rightful place in this world. Above all, this is a story about what I wish someone had told me those many years ago when my son was first diagnosed, and what I want mothers just beginning this journey with their autistic child to know.

Everything will be okay. Prayers will be answered, just not on the time line you're looking for. The poignant beauty of these children will open your heart and transform you as a person in ways you will never imagine. Trust in your personal judgments, ability, and power will be your biggest ally; pride is more powerful than shame.

Raising a child with autism is important work. Aside from your job of helping your child be his or her best self, you have another important responsibility: to be a role model of tolerance, compassion, and acceptance in a society all too inclined to judge and discount the disabled among us or those who are called different in any way. Gandhi is credited with saying, "you must be the change you want to see in the world."

Yes, raising a child with a disability is hard and exhausting. It's a marathon, not a sprint. But just as running cleared my head, autism opened my heart. While I will never know what Lee experiences inside his head, I do know we share a precious connection to the experience of humanity, to profound love, and to a life worth living.

CHAPTER 1:
THE PERFECT FAMILY

I grew up in the 1950s and 60s, formed by loving parents in a Catholic environment. Saturday weekly confession and Sunday mass were not an option but a commandment in our home. We were faithful in our obligations to our beliefs, whether it was having meatless Fridays or observing all Holy Days. We didn't read scriptures or pray outwardly, but it was a silent devotion that made a big impression on me.

My parents were a product of the Great Depression. Neither of them went beyond a ninth-grade education, but I never felt that they lacked intelligence. They were both hard working and they felt fortunate to work their jobs in the factories. My mother wanted to help my father provide for my two brothers and me, so she chose to work outside the home, which was unusual at that time. I was responsible for much of the housework, as my mother worked so many hours. We had what we needed in life. I was very content and appreciative for all they provided. More than the material objects were the feeling that all three of us siblings were loved. They trusted us, and encouraged us in school and with our sports. They were always there for us.

When the swimming pool was built in our community, it became my home away from home in the summer. I found my independence in those summer days. I spent hours and hours, either practicing with the swim team or hanging out with a fun group of school classmates. We laughed and laughed all the time, always enjoying each other's company. They are still my friends to this day.

Athletics were so important to me growing up, whether it was swimming, field hockey, or basketball. I loved everything about competition.

After graduation from high school, I went into the business world, trying to work my way up to a secretarial position.

My husband, John, and I met on a blind date in the fall of 1968 that was set up by a mutual friend. I was twenty, and he was handsome and older at twenty-six. We dated for seven months, got engaged, and then married in the fall of 1969. Young and in love, we had everything wonderful in life before us.

We came from two totally different backgrounds. John was one of nine children who lived on a farm in a nearby community. His family was German, dating back to the early days of Pennsylvania. I would say they were serious, hard-working people. They were a very tight-knit family, and they enjoyed themselves in a quiet manner in comparison to my gregarious, outgoing Polish family. We really were quite different from each other. We were opposites in many ways, but very much in love with each other. We've worked through many differences in parenting styles over the years, but one constant was our love and devotion to each other and our three sons.

We were blessed with our first son, Matthew John, in 1970. Intuitive with tremendous interest in the world around him, Matt performed all the baby firsts at a rapid rate. He walked by nine months old and he began talking by the age of one. We felt so joyful with our healthy, happy, little boy.

Increasing amounts of toys, baby clothing, and a toddler enjoying the new-found freedoms of walking required more room than our one-bedroom apartment could comfortably handle so we bought land in Robesonia, a small town in rural Pennsylvania, to build a home. Having just completed his journeyman electrician test, John worked hard during the day at his construction jobs and even harder in the evenings and weekends building our modest rancher in the country.

Life was wonderful. We moved ourselves and baby Matt into our partially finished home in the summer of 1971. Our country property felt so remote to me. We only had a few neighbors, who were separated from us by acres and acres of woods and farmland. I remember being startled awake the first morning in our new house by cows mooing outside the open window. John was raised on a farm and was used to the sounds of the countryside. He assured me that the cows were in the neighboring farmer's pasture, not outside our window. Our new home was in stark contrast to where I grew up, but I have since learned to love all the sights and sounds of country living.

With John away during the days working as an electrician, I stayed busy with the job of being a mom. I took up the hobby of sewing, both for enjoyment and necessity. Money was tight, so if I wanted curtains for the house or new clothing, I bought inexpensive material and made them myself. I also sewed items that were trending at the time, such as fabric wreaths, door draft stoppers, spice hangers, and pillows. I learned crewelwork, a surface embroidery using yarn, which I sold at craft shows to earn money for small purchases. I enjoyed doing these things when Matt was napping or when he was in bed for the night.

Likewise, lively Matt enjoyed all of the usual activities that little boys love: catching a ball, reading books, building with blocks, and playing with toy cars. He caught on to almost everything we presented to him. He was a very inquisitive little boy who needed a playmate.

I was blessed with another pregnancy when Matt was seventeen months old. My second pregnancy unfolded much like my first, bringing with it the usual morning sickness and weight gain. I felt the strain of dealing with pregnancy while already having a small child, but otherwise I felt quite normal. I watched my diet, took care of myself, and my pregnancy went full term without any problems. While sitting on the floor one evening, watching television, my water broke. We rushed to the hospital as my contractions grew closer and closer together. Within an hour and a half, to our delight, Lee Jonathan entered the world at 9:45 p.m. on April 5, 1973. Another precious little boy! We were ecstatic!

We loved and nurtured our new baby the same way we loved and nurtured his big brother, something that would later be disturbingly called into question. Naturally, I viewed my experience with my new baby through the lens of what I experienced with my firstborn. Unlike Matt as a newborn, Lee squirmed in my arms when I tried to cuddle and rock him to sleep. *How odd that he wouldn't let me rock him to sleep,* I thought, but he'd fall asleep on his own when I laid him in his crib and left him soothe himself to sleep. He didn't demand my attention the way his brother did. Rarely did he cry. He didn't draw attention to his discomforts, which made it difficult to know if he was hungry, had an upset stomach, needed a diaper change, or just needed love and attention.

As those first months ticked by, we waited anxiously for Lee to crawl, walk, speak, and play. Those milestones seemed to be taking longer for Lee than they did for his big brother or for his cousins who were the same age. I routinely questioned pediatricians about my concern. Lee was about four months old when he started getting ear infections, and we often ended up at the doctor for exams and medicine. I'd use the opportunity to also raise questions about his development, but the pediatricians at the practice kept telling me not to compare the boys. They told me that every child is different and reaches benchmarks on their own time. I tried to put it out of my mind. Watching nieces and nephews, who were the same ages as my boys, however, served as a regular reminder of the things Lee wasn't doing yet. I quietly monitored their progress, using it as a measuring stick for Lee's. It wasn't hard to see that Lee was very different. I worried, but had nothing concrete to do about it. We gave him the same love and attention we gave to his older brother, and hoped he would soon catch up in his own time.

As Lee grew into a toddler, he enjoyed when I sang his favorite nursery rhymes to him over and over again. He smiled and grunted for me to do it again and again. It was my connection with him, as I felt that there were only isolated times when I really felt the connection with him. He loved watching *Sesame Street* and *Captain Noah* on television with his big brother, but interestingly, I noticed the typical interaction between two brothers never occurred: no disagreements, no tug of war with their toys. The fact that Lee was too good actually began concerning me. Matt always tried to initiate play, but Lee never responded. So they played separately. I also noticed an unusual, distant look on Lee's face during the rare occasion when he made eye contact. When I was feeding him or repeatedly singing his favorite songs to him, he made eye contact, but otherwise Lee rarely looked at his family members with curiosity or interest in what we were doing.

Physically, Lee's limbs seemed limp and loose-jointed as he grew. Again, this was very unlike what I remembered his older brother's to be at a young age. He didn't sit up independently until seven or eight months; he failed to pull to standing until twelve months and only started walking at eighteen months, which was distressingly late. Until then, he bottom-scooted or commando crawled, using his arms to pull himself around on his belly and kicking his legs to push from behind. He'd take stairs sitting down. Despite practice, our toddler was unable to jump.

Working to help Lee walk, I noticed he never seemed interested in using any type of communication to ask for what he wanted. He would not vocalize to request a toy. He never crawled after an item that interested him and was content with whatever was given to him. He just waited patiently for whatever he was given. Most times, he was disinterested.

Lee didn't know basic words like over, under, in, and out. These are words a two-year-old should start to recognize, but we thought perhaps he was lagging because Matt always did things for him. Matt gave Lee some of his favorite toys for Lee to play with, hoping Lee would join him, but Lee chose to play alone. I noticed early on that Matt grew protective of Lee and attentive to his idiosyncrasies. Mostly, Lee made frequent, monotonous, semi-musical sounds with no intent to communicate anything. Lee was often inattentive to people who were speaking to him, and more tuned into the sounds around him like cars going by, the TV, or a radio playing. We tried unsuccessfully to get Lee to engage in reciprocal speech—the back-and-forth imitation of words and phrases. But he was able to recite the ABCs and parts of a television show or songs he had heard.

On one hand, this all seemed odd. Something wasn't quite right, but we couldn't put our fingers on what exactly was askew. On the other hand, this behavior was normal for Lee. A quiet, content personality, not a go-getter was just who he was. Nonetheless, I privately worried that something was wrong and signs that was indeed the case kept popping up in the course of everyday life.

Instead of playing with Matt's toy cars, driving them around as one would expect for a little boy, Lee placed them at eye level and moved them bit by bit to watch the wheels move ever so slowly. Never did he speed them up as other little boys did. He delighted in watching car wheels, or any-thing with wheels, spin around and around. He never stacked alphabet letter blocks. No matter what toy I placed before him, Lee always played with it in a way different from how it was intended.

Soon, I began observing Lee finding and examining angles—from telephone wires he'd spot while riding in the car, to the backs of chairs, tables, and even edges of walls when walking from one room to another.

At some point, he started to enjoy watching the hands of a clock go around. He simulated the clock physically by hold-ing his index finger, as someone would do to say their sport's team is number one. He'd then crisscross his index finger on his other hand to imitate the moving hands of a clock. He did this constantly. Walk into any room, he'd find the clock and position himself where he could watch it. It didn't take long before we had all the clocks and watches in our house covered or hidden, and we were covering the clocks when visiting family too. *Why did he find clocks so interesting?* I was puzzled and worried. *What could this be?*

With mounting concerns over Lee's development, I felt increasingly alone after John left for work each morning. It was solely up to me to dig in and try to make a difference for Lee. As a young mother, I took my job quite seriously, trying so hard to give my little boys proper nourishment and expose them to learning opportunities, stimulating events, and fun activities. At the same time, I tried with all my might to unlock what didn't seem right in Lee's world. I had a sinking, defeated feeling deep down that whatever I tried to do with Lee was not going to change who he was. I somehow sensed we were in this for the long haul.

At Sunday dinners with extended family, I'd routinely get asked how Lee was doing. I tried to cover up for his unusual behavior by saying he was just tired or sick or getting sick, all of which was true, as Lee's frequent ear infections were usually paired with cold symptoms such as a runny nose and a high fever. Taking Lee to the pediatrician grew increasingly common and these visits came with lots of antibiotics and cough medicine that made his eyes glaze over. Of course, Lee being sick wasn't the whole truth, so I'd attempt to deflect the situation entirely by changing the subject or drawing attention to my nieces, nephews, and other children in the room. Obviously, however, something was wrong. The growth and development of young cousins close to Lee's age served as a painful reminder he was not making the progress he should be. Increasingly, my own home became the only place I felt comfortable and able to relax. Most places I learned to put up my guard, ready to defend my precious little boy.

Day in and day out, I prayed Lee would wake up and be a normal little boy, but every morning when that didn't happen, I was disappointed. Most every day, I'd call my mother for encouragement and advice on getting through the day without worrying. "Say your prayers," she'd always say.

CHAPTER 2:

"IS HE RETARDED?"

One early summer day in 1976, when Lee was three years old, I went grocery shopping with the boys and my mother-in-law, Anna. On the way out of the supermarket, with my cart full of groceries and the boys in tow, my mother-in-law turned to me and mentioned that the cashier asked her if Lee was retarded. "Of course, he's not retarded!" I snapped. "How could she ask such a question?"

I didn't ask at the time, but I doubt my mother-in-law responded to the clerk in defense of Lee. As a woman born in 1912 and living on a rural farm, she probably didn't feel comfortable engaging in conversation with others, especially strangers. Looking back over the years, I think women her age didn't feel that they had a voice or the empowerment that women experience today. I imagine she would have had difficulty defending Lee because she more than likely had the same question as the cashier. She wasn't at all familiar with anyone in her family having unusual behaviors of any kind.

Driving in silence, I held back my tears until I dropped off my mother-in-law at her home. Then, alone in the car with the boys, I quietly cried the rest of the way home. I couldn't understand why someone would ask such a question. At the time, I was already self-conscious about Lee's behaviors. He sometimes held his hands over his ears and whined to himself. His aloofness was obvious to others. I waited anxiously for John to come home from work that day, and I tearfully told him what had happened. He couldn't believe a total stranger would say such a thing. Neither John nor I had experience dealing with issues of mental illness, and we both struggled with worry over what could be wrong with Lee. We decided to take more active steps in order to determine what exactly was going on with our precious, but puzzling, little boy. From that moment, we had to forge our own path for Lee.

After infancy, the boys made routine visits every year to our area children's clinic for their wellness pediatrician appointments, usually rotating with one of the clinic's different doctors. These visits felt like a struggle, because the doctors never suggested that anything was wrong with Lee. They all took a hands-off approach. They kept giving Lee his inoculations, but never questioned me about his behavior and never offered suggestions or support when I mentioned concerns. It was all business as usual. No one ever said Lee wasn't perfect. We were told Lee was a very special child and we were sent on our way with mounting worry and doubt. We knew by the looks of questioning family members that they didn't agree that Lee was just special. Quite honestly, deep down, we didn't believe it either, but we were afraid of what we might learn.

After the incident at the grocery store, I became frantic. I scheduled an immediate appointment with the pediatrician. I pressed the issue of his delayed speech and motor development and received a referral to a child psychologist.

Well-respected in the pediatric community, the doctor was in her mid-forties or early fifties, with short, curly brown hair. Her casual dress gave me the impression she didn't worry too much about her appearance. She had a calming voice with soothing mannerisms and she began our late-June appointment by carefully interviewing John and me about our concerns. She wanted to know about Lee's medical history in addition to our family and living situation, along with our social habits. She noted in her exam report: "The family lives in what Mrs. Ruth describes as 'total isolation' on two acres near Robesonia. There are no other children in the area." *Why would she underline this statement in an effort to emphasize it? Why was she concerned about living in a rural area? How did our home's location relate to Lee's behaviors?* I wondered.

She also took Lee aside for a thorough physical and neurological examination, measuring his weight, height, and head circumference. She took his pulse and checked his neck, thyroid, chest, belly, genitals, spine, skin, arms, and legs. She left no stone unturned in her examination. She attempted to elicit speech and observed him at play.

"Lee is an unusual child with mild delay in all areas of development," read her final analysis. "His responses today arouse suspicion of a high-frequency hearing loss. Many of his deficiencies in fine motor skills have a dystonic quality consisting of sporadic movements. He certainly has many signs of neurological immaturity. Much of his behavior suggests a tendency toward volitional withholding, and this may be a factor in his slow speech."

As follow-up, she recommended we have Lee's hearing tested, consult a speech therapist concerning language stimulation, and have a complete psychological evaluation by a highly-skilled child psychologist. Before leaving our appointment she said, "Lee doesn't need to speak at this time. He could make his way to New York and back without talking." *How bizarre and unhelpful to frame my son's behavior like that,* I thought. I left the appointment with more questions than answers. I didn't have the courage to question authority, so I began following through with her recommendations.

I made arrangements with a friend of our family who was an audiologist at the Reading Hospital. Lee was fearful of the equipment and the soundproof room where his hearing was tested. Lee also didn't understand the audiologist's directions such as "Put your finger up if you hear this sound," so it was difficult to test accurately as a result. The audiologist was also trying to observe Lee's eye movements in an attempt to observe when he heard sounds, but Lee's whining and behavior couldn't validate accurate results. The results of that test were inconclusive.

John was not in favor of Lee seeing another psychologist. He seemed to have a hard time admitting that Lee might have a mental illness. John was much more deliberate than I was. He had an ability to stand back and observe a situation before reacting to it. I, on the other hand, felt panicked and needed to act immediately. Slow and steady as opposed to fast and impulsive. Perhaps John thought Lee's symptoms would eventually work out in their own time or that disabilities happen to other people's children, other families. I felt bewildered by what the mental-health community was telling us, yet instinctively I knew something wasn't right with Lee. Fear, confusion, denial, an awful cocktail of all three—something drove us to keep searching for answers and pursue the psychologist's recommendations.

While the barrage of evaluations all happened within just a few weeks, the answers to our questions seemed to take an eternity. I had no idea how long the process would take. I unknowingly believed this was going to be a quick fix. In the meantime, we focused on the one thing we could control: loving Lee and treating him the same way we treated his big brother, Matt. I continued to hug and kiss him as much as I did Matt. Not a day went by that I did not cuddle with him and sing lullabies to him. He squirmed in my arms and I can't say he enjoyed this time, but I did it anyway. I massaged his body with sweet-smelling baby lotion after his daily bath. I was trying to unlock the door to my son's problem, but I was unable to find the key.

Eventually, I convinced John to agree to a complete psychological evaluation for Lee. We made an appointment at the Berks County Intermediate Unit (BCIU) with a highly recognized child psychologist. The psychologist was a slightly built man who commanded the room as though he were much taller. He was impeccably dressed, giving me the impression that he paid attention to detail. I felt comfortable with him as he talked and tried to play with Lee. I felt that he had his suspicions about the nature of Lee's problems, as he suggested we make an appointment with a child psychiatrist in the Reading area. With his gentle voice the psychologist assured us that we would get help for our son.

A few more days went by until we obtained an appointment with a psychiatrist. My first impression of this doctor was quite different. He appeared disorganized as he walked into the room. He wore a plaid sport coat, a mismatched tie and shirt, and brown pants. How funny that I remember that so vividly. He was in his fifties, with dark, graying hair styled in a college cut, a hairstyle typically worn by much younger men.

He had no smile and came across as very matter of fact, giving us only information with no emotion.

Both professionals took Lee into a play-room where they evaluated him by showing him simple picture cards and asking him to do certain tasks that were considered age appropriate. After what seemed like a very long time, John and I were called back into the room. We sat with the doctors around a tiny children's table. From behind his horn-rimmed glasses, the psychiatrist looked us in the eyes and said, "Lee is autistic." "He's artistic?" I asked. "No," he replied. "He's autistic. I recommend you put him in an institution. I know a few in Philadelphia that I can recommend."

After he mentioned the institution, I went blank and didn't hear another word that was said at that meeting. John and I sat dumbfounded and devastated on kid-sized chairs in the preschool therapy room with our young son, trying to grasp what we had just been told.

Who puts a three-year-old child in an institution? Were they crazy? Did they have a heart? Did someone say my perfect little boy wasn't perfect? How can these people be so cruel? They couldn't mean what they were saying. The psychologist gave us a box of tissues to wipe our tears. The psychiatrist showed no empathy and made no attempt to console us. The meeting ended with John and me leaving in a daze.

We drove away in silent disbelief to pick up Matt at my mother's house. I worried about how I could look my mother in the eyes and tell her that her grandson, who she adored, wasn't perfect. And how could I also tell her that I was pregnant with our third child?

CHAPTER 3:
QUICK CURE?

Lee's diagnosis landed in July 1976, the U.S. Bicentennial. Parades and celebrations passed me by as I stood on the sidelines with a heavy heart and worried mind, devastated and consumed by the news that our son had some sort of strange disability. Our ordinary young family suddenly looked tragically different. Our dreams for the future felt that they were being ripped away.

Before Lee's diagnosis, each day felt like a struggle living in confusion and concern, waiting in nervous anticipation for one of our pediatricians to say something about Lee's condition that would give us clarity and direction so that we could help him get better and move on with normal family life. But awareness of autism in the early 1970s was minimal and information didn't exist, at least not within my little circle of contacts: my community, family, friends, doctors, acquaintances, teachers, and no one mentioned autism. It just wasn't a word that ever came up in conversation. No one knew how to help, and no one offered to help either.

There was no Internet. I couldn't Google "autism" and connect to the autism website. There was no National Autism Awareness Month, and there were no autism support groups. All we knew was that we were on our own in our day-to-day dealings with a very complicated little boy.

It seemed to me that only a handful of specialists had a sense of what was going on in the treatment of autism. When one of them finally gave Lee the autism diagnosis, it came out of nowhere and landed on us like a ton of bricks. "Careful what you wish for," the saying goes. After years of praying for answers to Lee's problems, we had a new daily struggle: curing our son's autism, a phenomenon we didn't even understand.

Dazed and uncertain of what to do, we found ourselves thrust into early childhood intervention, which consisted of art therapy, speech therapy, occupational therapy, and a special preschool class for autistic children. It was the only one of its kind in Berks County at the time.

Occupational therapy at Easter Seals was our first treatment experience for Lee. Easter Seals provided a range of services to children living with disabilities, but there weren't many, if any, other autistic children there at the time. One little boy that we met at our therapy sessions was about five years old and had Muscular Dystrophy. He started to stumble and lose mobility after having no problems previously. He progressed to crutches and then to a wheel chair. It was devastating to watch this little boy try to cope with such a debilitating problem. The rest of the children were severely disabled, which I found deeply traumatic against the rawness of Lee's jarring diagnosis only a few weeks earlier. Other than my life with Lee, this was my first time being exposed to what disabilities could look like and it frightened me. I had never before been exposed to so many little children with so many challenges.

We were introduced to a kind and talented occupational therapist referred to as Miss Joyce. Each week, Miss Joyce welcomed Lee with a big hug and smile before escorting him to the therapy room where she'd guide him through therapy designed to kick-start the areas of his brain that might not be working properly. For example, she'd spin him in a hammock to watch for the nystagmus in his eyes, looking for him to be dizzy. Interestingly, Lee didn't get dizzy. His therapist explained to me this was because Lee has an underdeveloped vestibular system. Therapeutic swings provide vestibular stimulation to individuals with sensory-processing issues. The back-and-forth motion helps to calm overstimulated children, improve balance, and develop important motor skills. She worked on other skills, trying to get Lee's limp body to be more secure. *Where was the disconnection?* I wondered. Lee continued receiving therapy at Easter Seals for many years, faithfully leaving school and getting his therapy weekly. We tried to continue some of the exercises that were introduced to him at home on off days. He received a sit and spin as a gift so that we could mimic the swing used with Miss Joyce.

Since we immediately rejected the institution for our son, it was recommended that Lee move forward with a preschool for autistic children. There was only one preschool class designated for children with mental disabilities in our county at the time. Our school district did not have any accommodations, so Lee had to travel thirty minutes away to a half-day preschool that accommodated autistic children. His preschool teachers were my first contact with professionals who knew more than most people about autism. Lee was one of eight children in the class, all of whom seemed to have varying degrees of autism. Some of them were a few years older than Lee. There were three girls. The school district bused him during the school year, while I provided transportation in the summer months. Luckily, the public education system paid for his schooling. Once again, with raw emotions, I struggled to see Lee in class among mentally disabled children. He spent two years at this preschool.

During each class, Lee went through a routine of singing, speech therapy, exercise, and occupational therapy. The teachers tried to get the children outside every day, taking a walk around the school grounds or just playing on the playground. Everyone involved in his learning showed our unusual little boy genuine care and affection. Lee, however, seemed detached from all of the attention he was given. He'd cover his ears with his hands as if the sounds of daily living disturbed him. He'd whine aloud, perhaps his way of coping and talking himself through a world he didn't understand. It was explained to me that Lee didn't know where he was in his space. He didn't understand that his limbs attached to his body. He didn't know how to interact with other people. In fact, he didn't understand much about the world around him, as if a thick cloud surrounded him.

I was on the edge of my seat each day, eagerly waiting to learn about Lee's progress in school. I remember the banner day when I picked Lee up from preschool and his teachers were elated to report that Lee spoke words. It wasn't conversation, but rather he identified objects on picture cards. I, too, was thrilled to see gains in his development, even though Lee at the age of three was just learning words Matt had learned at a much younger age. The difference in skills between my two boys was striking. Rarely was Lee's speech spontaneous;

it almost always had to be coached. Matt, exhibited such quickness in learning, while everything seemed to be such a struggle for Lee. Even Lee's physical health was increasingly becoming a struggle, saddled with reoccurring ear infections that left him sick nearly every month.

In addition to enrolling Lee in this special preschool, we followed up on the doctor's recommendation to pursue art therapy. I wasn't sure what art therapy would be about, but I dutifully followed through as suggested.

On his first day of art therapy, Lee was introduced to an art therapist who was very kind and gentle with him. He asked Lee to draw a picture of himself. When Lee didn't respond to his request, the therapist drew a circle on the paper. He prodded Lee to draw the eyes, nose, mouth, and ears on the paper. Lee took the crayon and initially used it to imitate a clock. There was a bit of silence and then I encouraged Lee to draw on the circle. He could not respond. He colored a bit on the outside of the circle and then stopped. That abruptly ended his first attempt at art therapy.

The art therapist then escorted us into an adjoining room for discussion with a new psychologist, who started asking questions related to how I felt about Lee. Did I cuddle him or did I ignore him? I always affirmed with enthusiasm how much I loved Lee and that he was a wanted pregnancy. I had a strange feeling that I needed to prove myself to this doctor.

CHAPTER 4:
WHO'S TO BLAME?

When John came home from work, I shared the day's developments from Lee's appointment. Early in our experience with art therapy, John commented on how many of the doctor's questions pertained to what I did or how I treated Lee. "It sounds like the psychologist is analyzing you," he said.

I didn't think much of this until our next session when the psychologist introduced me to the refrigerator mom theory. He said lack of maternal warmth causes autism and Lee's withdrawal represents an act of turning away to seek comfort from cold, emotionless, detached care-giving. He explained where Lee's autism developed from: Me.

"Me? That can't be! We live in a loving family. I love and treat Lee the same as my other son, who is developing just fine," I replied. I explained how I wanted to and tried cuddling Lee, but he squirmed and fussed and cried until I'd put him down and then he immediately settled. I just thought Lee didn't like that. How could I be stifling his development?

He watched me intently as he listened, trying to read me, trying to determine if I was being truthful.

Crushed and utterly defeated, I sobbed uncontrollably all the way home. I followed through with only a few more art-therapy sessions after that incident. Having Lee in a room drawing pictures with an art therapist while this psychologist analyzed me clearly did nothing to help my child. While the psychologist may have had the credentials that he felt empowered him to scrutinize my failings, he offered no suggestions to help us move forward to help Lee. John and I quickly determined that we were terminating art therapy, hoping our money could be invested in services that would have more productive results for Lee.

The emotional pain I experienced at the time the refrigerator mom theory was presented to me was overwhelming. I still reeled with the fear and confusion from having my precious son being diagnosed with a disability. To be accused of not nurturing my child and told that I wasn't a loving parent and that was the reason my child didn't respond to me and other people devastated me. *How could this professional say something that hurtful to me as I desperately sought his help to find a cure for my child's problem?* I wondered.

Scared, perplexed, and only a few months into Lee's diagnosis, I didn't understand anything about autism. I yearned to know how to make Lee's world better. To question my love for Lee, the only thing I felt certain about, was crushing. Questioning my self-worth, I sank deeper into a painful sense of guilt that Lee was paying the price for something I did wrong.

At night, I'd lay awake wondering how this happened and what I could have done differently. Maybe I wasn't spending enough time playing with and teaching him. Perhaps I worked with and played more with Matt than Lee.

Lee was a very easy-going baby. He didn't cry out nor was he demanding. He never had a tantrum. He really was happiest when left to play alone in the way that was comforting to him. Maybe I should have demanded his attention. Maybe I ate the wrong foods during pregnancy. I stayed away completely from nitrates during my first pregnancy, but perhaps got a bit careless while pregnant with Lee. Why didn't I realize earlier how important eye contact was, and instead I assumed Lee was watching his family members? I questioned everything, all while six months pregnant with my third child. Every night after my boys were asleep, I prayed Lee would improve and be a changed little boy in the morning. I trusted we'd find a cure.

Nonetheless, I refused to accept a diagnosis of autism. A number of professionals we interacted with characterized Lee as having "autistic tendencies." I remembered being introduced to the phrase "developmentally delayed." For a long time, I'd tell people Lee was just developmentally delayed with some autistic tendencies. This sounded much more hopeful to me. I placed my confidence in curing Lee on the assumption he wasn't really autistic in the first place, even though he met the criteria: lack of eye contact, lack of meaningful speech, lack of social interaction, lack of smiling or reciprocal facial gestures. He had them all. In public, I started deflecting attention away from Lee by quickly changing the subject, interjecting questions that would get people talking about themselves and their family instead of me and mine. No one likes to feel different, and I didn't either.

I began channeling my fear and worry into research, desperately trying to understand Lee's experience living with autism. I visited the library and read any book or article I could find on the subject. If I stumbled upon a reference on TV or in a waiting-room magazine article, I'd try to track down more information. If I read about a special diet for Lee, I'd try it. If I heard about a therapy or behavior modification that didn't require a trained specialist, I'd try it. The only way to prove the validity of methods and theories I came across was to test them myself with Lee.

Once, I experimented with using treats as incentive for appropriate behavior. If Lee did something I asked him to do such as "Put the button in the box," I gave him a treat. I didn't understand that Lee didn't have the capacity to make associations, so he just kept looking for the treats, not realizing that I was asking him to accomplish a task first. Without any expertise or guidelines to compare these approaches to, I winged it. Despite feeling I was conducting these therapies using the wrong methods; my best judgment was all I could trust.

Once I read about a mother who isolated herself in the bathroom with her autistic son. Every day, she stayed in the bathroom with her child for hours, forcing the child to give her eye contact and follow her commands. While it sounded promising, Lee wasn't my only child. I felt limited in what I could do and I had to be realistic. Who would care for my other little boy? In addition to Matt, I was pregnant. Helping Lee couldn't come at the cost of hurting Matt's development or that of my soon-to-be newborn. I would never compromise their needs in that way. I continued doing the best I could, searching for a cure, always hoping the situation would get easier.

When I was six months pregnant, I learned about a conference nearby of doctors discussing the rarity of autism and I decided to attend. By chance, I came upon the psychiatrist who had diagnosed Lee six months earlier. I greeted him cordially. He took one look at me and said, "I can't believe you're pregnant!" He was visibly disgusted. "Do you know what the chances of having another child like Lee or worse are?" he questioned. I just stood there, speechless and shattered. *How could this man be so cruel to me twice, first suggesting I send my vulnerable toddler to an institution and now this?* And no, I didn't know what my chances of having another child with autism were because I didn't understand anything that was happening to Lee. I didn't understand anything about autism, which was tearing away at my beautiful family. I felt like I was living in a nightmare.

Until that point, I never considered that my next baby could have the same problems as Lee. Matt didn't have any problems, so I assumed Lee's situation was random with no connection to heredity. DNA and genetics were not topics of conversation at that time in the 1970s. I lived in silent fear for my unborn baby. Hearing those words, telling me how great the chances were of our baby becoming autistic, constantly replayed in my mind. My anxiety and worry grew along with the baby inside me. As my mother had taught me, I prayed for God to give me strength. *Oh God, please hear my prayers.*

CHAPTER 5:
OUR ATTEMPT AT NORMAL

I always dreamed of having a large family, possibly six children. I knew I had enough love in my heart to share. The reality of Lee's situation, however, combined with the cost of raising children and the additional expense of helping a special-needs child modified those dreams. Our health insurance covered none of the costs, we were quickly learning. In the delivery room while holding our third precious child, I felt relieved, blessed, and content with our beautiful three sons.

William David, a strong name, I thought. With Billy's delivery, I processed the moments without panic. I felt confident we'd be okay. I also felt certain Lee's autism would soon be corrected. Billy's birth was relaxed, and not nearly as instantaneous as Lee's birth. We didn't know in advance we were going to be blessed with another little boy until I saw him emerge and the doctor announced, "It's a boy!" The exhilaration was overwhelming. Crying tears of happiness I remember saying, "How will I mother three boys?" John responded jokingly that I could join them when they go hunting. "Who me, go hunting?" I responded joyfully.

I was so happy to bring our third son home to our small house in the country. The theme song from *My Three Sons*, a popular sitcom at the time, played and danced in my mind for months and months after Billy was born. Three boys! I was truly ecstatic. As the early weeks with baby Billy ticked by, any lingering worry from my public shaming over my baby's chances of being autistic increasingly faded from my mind. I watched vigilantly for eye contact or small indicators of something other than normal. Billy enjoyed being cuddled and rocked. He was a pleasant and easy-going child, yet he'd let me know when he was tired or hungry or when he needed his diaper changed. Unlike his brother Lee, Billy certainly put me on notice. At about four weeks old came Billy's monumental first smile! I cried tears of happiness once again! My newborn was developing beautifully and I could channel that nervous energy back to Lee, hoping I could transform him to be a very shiny light.

Having three young children certainly had me stepping, but motherhood felt wonderful even as I found my days busier than ever before, getting Matt ready for school and taking care of two other little boys who both needed so much attention. Because Lee was quiet and didn't make his needs known like his baby brother, I intentionally measured my time wisely between both of them, ensuring each child got equal attention while Matt was away at school.

Little Billy was a wonderful addition to our family in so many ways. He added so much joy to our family! He enhanced our many car rides to Lee's doctors, schools, and therapies. Because of our location, our trips all required at least a thirty-minute drive each direction. This meant disrupting Billy's naps, mealtimes, and playtimes to jump back in the car for yet another appointment. Easy-going and pleasant, Billy never seemed to mind. He had a smile for everyone we met and ate up all the attention from caring therapists who'd fuss over him. He was also just as happy to content himself with his toys. He seemed to love all the new experiences, and having him along seemed to lighten the otherwise heavy energy surrounding all of Lee's treatments.

Pondering what I could do to help Lee learn in a normal environment without any other children with mental challenges, I decided to experiment with Lee's education when he was in the second year of his special education. I enrolled him in a normal preschool program two afternoons a week. I felt like I needed to take some control of Lee's education, which I valued so much. Lee was five, while the other children were younger. I wanted him to socialize and see how other children played. I didn't understand the degree of difficulty he had relating to other people at this time, I only knew my instincts were telling me to find some place Lee could be with other children his age who talked normally, who could show him how to interact through play. Since Matt was at elementary school and Billy was still a young toddler, I wanted to fill that gap and provide Lee with exposure to children his age with normal behaviors rather than just those in the remedial learning environment. *Maybe he'd absorb and mirror that behavior,* I reasoned.

With Billy in tow, I faithfully picked up Lee on Tuesdays and Fridays at lunch-time at his special school and took him to a traditional preschool in a neighboring town. It was a private school, operating from September to June, inside of a church. I valued the Christian setting it provided. Private meant its tuition added another expense for John to absorb in our budget, along with the costs of Lee's early intervention treatments, which were not covered by our health insurance.

The head teacher had a heart of gold and an amazingly caring personality common to so many elementary school teachers. She appeared to truly believe she could make a difference with Lee. She included him in singing, storytelling, answering questions, and the same activities she used to teach and engage the other children in the class, but she struggled to gain Lee's cooperation.

A number of times, I'd stalk the school to spy on his class outside at recess or free play. As all the other children played together, Lee stood off alone in his own world, ignoring the other children and looking at different angles on the playground. My heart broke. It was painfully obvious that placing Lee in a class of normal children wasn't giving him the outcome I was praying for, and I grew increasingly concerned how Lee's need for additional attention affected the other children who deserved the teacher's attention as well. I didn't want her to feel compelled to spend so much time with Lee to take away from the other children, and I didn't enroll him for a second year.

CHAPTER 6:
ILLNESS AS A CAUSE OR AS A SYMPTOM?

Further complicating Lee's learning was his health, which continued to cycle up and down every four to six weeks. Typically, Lee only felt well a week or two out of that time period. Like spotting subtle signs of changing seasons, I could tell when he was starting to decline. Dark circles formed under his eyes, his energy would tank, and then he'd be hit with ear infections and high fevers. You can't send a child to school with a fever and runny nose, so I'd have to keep him home from the education he desperately needed at such an important time in his childhood. We visited the pediatrician and were prescribed medicines, containing artificial colorings and flavorings, which made his eyes glaze over and fogged his brain on top of what autism already clouded. There was discussion at that time that these additions to children's medicines were causing various reactions to certain children who were consuming them. I definitely saw a change in Lee when he consumed these syrups. Lee's pediatricians didn't investigate the causes of his frequent illnesses, and I didn't speak out about it either. I was so unsure of all that was going on with Lee's mental and physical development, I just didn't know what to do. I was baffled and felt even more alone as to what to do to help this sad little boy who was definitely in a world of his own.

One day, as I looked at Lee's preschool class picture, the severity of his poor health hit me. Despite the adorable steel-blue sweater and matching pants I put on him for fall photo day, he looked terrible. He looked so sad. He looked like a sickly, troubled, little boy. It scared me to think his problems were so complicated.

Lee's frequent illnesses stole my attention away from finding help for his development. His pediatricians didn't see a link between his physical health and his mental health. I was trying hard to understand the dilemma we were in, but didn't know how to get us out. I didn't know who to contact or where to go for help, other than what I could gather from people and doctors we already were in contact with. I tried to listen to other mothers at play-groups. Living in a small, rural town in the 1970s, I only had access to what was in front of me, what was in my immediate circle of family, friends, and community of acquaintances, and none of them had ever experienced dealing with an autistic child.

I struggled under the toll of worrying about Lee and keeping up with the demands of caring for three young children. I cried to any family member who would listen, though most seemed reluctant to get involved. I could always count on my mother to listen and be with me when I cried, but I also recognized the helplessness she was feeling as a grandmother dealing with her grandson's problems. She kept Lee's situation private, never sharing with anyone that he had difficulties. She frequently talked to her sisters on the phone, but no one from our extended family knew what was going on because none of us ever said anything about it out loud. She knew Lee was different, but she refused to admit it, long after I did, that he was autistic. She always found a twist to explain Lee's behaviors. My mother would just say he had a problem or that it took Lee a little longer to complete a task, but she never referred to him as disabled or mentioned Lee in a negative voice. She always saw the positive in Lee. Her background and social circle were much more limited than mine, and she wasn't a reader or a researcher. She placed her trust in me that I would do the best job to get to the bottom of Lee's problem. "Everything will work out," she said so many times. "Keep saying your prayers." I knew she always had my back no matter what, but I often guarded her from my pain because my pain became her pain. A mother knows her child, so she would immediately know I wasn't okay if we were together in person. When I talked to her on the phone, however, I often lied and said everything was fine.

The truth was I felt hopeless so much of the time. I was trying so hard, but didn't feel I was making a dent in the problem. I attempted to journal, but that fell off amid everything else I juggled. After the boys were tucked in bed for the night, I withdrew into my bedroom for a few minutes to pray and gather myself so I could regain control to deal with the hectic life I needed to somehow grow accustomed to. John coped differently. He could escape to work and be with other men. I felt so alone in how I was going to get through this. I tried to keep a smile on my face, but underneath I was in turmoil. I tried to take each day, one day at a time.

During this early time of searching, I somehow became aware of Dr. Eugene Shippen, a holistic doctor who practiced in the town where I grew up and where my parents still resided. Dr. Shippen was different from most doctors at the time. He believed in taking natural approaches before conventional medicines and he could evaluate Lee's complete health picture rather than just take care of medical needs such as colds. He had a gentle nature and was an open-minded, analytical, positive thinker who became an important part of a support team I didn't realize I was building.

Over the next thirty-six years, Dr. Shippen worked and experimented with different treatments and tests for Lee. He truly was trying to unlock this stubborn door. In hindsight, so much of it was a long shot. However, we always felt he was trying to find something that might make a difference.

Dr. Shippen ordered an array of tests, one of which included blood work for cytotoxic testing. This process of analyzing blood samples for allergies associated with food was performed in Nyack, New York. Our family drove Lee to this lab where the test was performed. In the 1970s, this was thought to be a reliable test, but in the following years, the theory has been debunked.

Lee also had a hair analysis to evaluate his hair for toxic minerals that might be impeding his learning and behavior. As usual, our insurance covered none of these tests, but John came up with the money to pay the bills because we wouldn't dare pass up an opportunity that could potentially help our little boy.

With each new test, we always thought we were on the verge of solving the mystery of Lee's behavior. Unfortunately, all of the testing did little to help us find an antidote to Lee's autism, but it did lead to what felt like the first shred of progress in my quest to help Lee since his diagnosis years earlier.

It turned out Lee suffered allergies to many foods: mainly wheat, chocolate, peanuts, milk, and eggs, all of which were staples of his diet. He loved bread, cheese, pasta, pudding, and ice cream. We needed to eliminate these and all the foods for which Lee tested positive.

Lee was placed on a rotation diet, which limited him to one food from each food group for an entire day. The foods we could include were only the foods that Lee did not test positive for allergies. That meant, for example, one day would consist only of chicken, rice, green beans, and peaches. The next day for breakfast, lunch, and dinner, the menu consisted of beef, oats, peas, and apples. I varied the way the food was prepared, but each day's designated foods were the only ones he was allowed to eat for the entire day. I kept a daily log as to how he behaved and reported back to Dr. Shippen.

Fortunately, I enjoyed cooking so I got creative. I turned oatmeal, which Lee didn't like the consistency of, into a crispy, golden, nutritious breakfast by frying it like a pancake. Sometimes I'd flavor the oatcakes with applesauce and cinnamon. Since Lee was allergic to cow's milk, I found a farm near our home that sold goat's milk. I used it in his cooking and I put it in the freezer with a little vanilla mixed in and scraped the frozen goat's milk into a dish for Lee's evening treat. He loved it! He didn't seem to notice the goat milk's icy consistency or the peculiar taste. He thought he was eating ice cream!

After eliminating all of the problem foods from his diet, Lee's physical health improved dramatically. When I think back, his health problems began around the same time I introduced him to solid foods. He was probably allergic from the start, but none of Lee's pediatricians ever mentioned allergies as a possibility. Instead, they just treated his symptoms with cold medicines that dulled his senses and were full of colorings and flavorings that likely further fed his allergies. By changing his diet, the dark circles under his eyes diminished, and he stopped getting the ear infections and colds every month. Not being sick, he could attend school more often and seemed better able to focus, both of which meant he was better equipped to learn. It wasn't the miracle cure for autism we were looking for, but it certainly eased the burden by not having to deal with illnesses all the time. This victory with his health also gave us a shred of optimism for progress in his mental development.

Dr. Shippen's devotion to helping Lee went beyond uncovering allergies. He and his staff welcomed Lee with open arms and gave me something I desperately needed at that time: empathy. Up until then, most of my encounters with pediatricians, psychologists, and doctors left me feeling alone, confused, guilty, or all three. Dr. Shippen, however, emerged as a much-needed blessing, routinely giving me little doses of hope during a time when feelings of frustration over helping Lee almost always ran high. Just when I felt as if there was nothing left to try to help Lee, Dr. Shippen would enter the exam room with a smile and new idea. Forward thinking, he seemed as much in a quest for solutions and prioritizing Lee's progress as I was, listening to my concerns, never saying anything to assign blame. If he had any doubts about positive outcomes for Lee, he never made them known to me. I felt heard, validated, and supported. He'd always give me as much time in our appointment as we needed, never rushing us out the door. In those early years of Lee's diagnosis, Dr. Shippen gained my trust in guiding my son's well-being, and I owe him much gratitude.

At the same time as I was dealing with Lee and his challenges, Matt's elementary school was planning to reduce the physical-education classes because of budget reasons. I began contemplating the connection between physical health and learning. I realized that the reason Lee was going to Easter Seals was to improve his gross motor skills, which would in turn help his overall learning. I made the assumption that this was also true for all children, and I was concerned about the negative impact this decision would have, not only on Matt, but all children.

A public hearing was held at the school's auditorium where teachers, school board members, and parents were invited to attend. The auditorium was packed with concerned individuals. As I listened to the discussions, Lee's experiences at Easter Seals kept coming to my mind and how the two skills were connected.

I felt compelled to speak out. I didn't grow up around empowered women who spoke out and shared their opinions, but I felt I had to be heard. I stood up in front of the assembly and voiced my concerns that children who were struggling with their gross motor skills might be unduly impacted by the elimination of teachers in physical education, thus impacting their fine motor skills and learning.

Nervously and with a shaky voice, I introduced myself and spoke about this connection. After speaking, relieved and satisfied with my comments, I sat down. Unbelievably, the Superintendent of Schools admitted to the audience that he wasn't listening and he asked me to repeat my concern. I then arose to repeat it all over again. I sat down again to applause from several teachers and parents. It was my first experience at public speaking and speaking my mind, but not the last. Regardless of the outcome, I felt that my voice was heard.

I believe in hindsight that this was the beginning of my advocacy for my children. It gave me the confidence to stand up to doctors and other professionals in my dealings with getting the help Lee needed and deserved.

CHAPTER 7:

SCHOOL'S IN SESSION

As Lee aged out of preschool, it was now time to enter full-day classes. The school district in which we resided did not have a special education class for autistic children, so Lee was bused to a nearby school district. He found himself with several of his classmates from preschool as well as other older children who were also autistic. There were twelve children in the class with various degrees of disability. As this was more than forty years ago, I am sure there are now many classes for autistic children with teachers who are wonderful and knowledgeable in their methods. For that I am thankful.

Lee's first-grade experience took him to Sinking Spring Elementary School. There, he was met by an energetic teacher, Sally Koch. She was the early elementary autistic teacher for the Berks County Intermediate Unit (BCIU), which is an educational service agency that provides a wide range of services to at-risk students and students with disabilities in our county. The BCIU was an umbrella service for special education, which included academic learning and psychological testing. These services were not economical or practical for districts to provide themselves.

Ms. Koch was wonderful with her students. She presented a bright and cheery demeanor. I was so appreciative of her caring and understanding. She worked with Lee on all the fundamental skills other children in normal elementary classes focused on learning. Lee's rate of success, however, proved minimal. It became apparent to me that a basic ability to communicate, something Lee didn't possess, held the key to most learning. Lee struggled with comprehension and retention.

For example, Lee couldn't understand that when he saw a piece of candy or a chewed piece of gum on the ground that he was not supposed to pick it up and eat it. He also picked up other items to eat. He ate ice incessantly. We often caught him picking up little pieces of paper he'd find on the ground and eating them. We had to diligently watch everything around us because we were never sure what would catch his eye and then go into his mouth. When he saw someone discard a food item, he did not demonstrate any recall from previous lessons about the danger of putting it into his mouth. Pica is a disorder that causes people to eat items that have no nutritional value. I learned years later that this odd behavior often occurs in people with severe developmental disabilities. The skills Lee learned in early elementary school were many skills that required constant reinforcement throughout his life.

Not all of Lee's education met my approval. When he was equivalent to the age for sixth grade, Lee was separated from his regular class, as many of the older students moved on to a junior high class. Lee was railroaded into an emotional-support classroom. No longer did he have a teacher like Ms. Koch who specialized in autism and its related challenges. Lee's class now was noisy, disorganized, and chaotic much of the time.

On one of the days that I picked Lee up for a therapy appointment, I walked into the classroom where many of the students were actually sailing paper airplanes at each other. I was certain that this was not the right classroom for Lee and I requested an IEP meeting with his teachers.

As required by the Education for All Handicapped Children's Act of 1975, all children who qualify for special education in any form require an Individual Education Plan or IEP. The IEP is developed by the education team for each child and indicates how each child's education will be customized in order to best serve them. It outlines specific goals for each student.

When I sat down for the meeting, Lee's teacher actually told me that he did not have an IEP for Lee. I couldn't believe my ears. I left that meeting abruptly with concerns regarding the quality of education, or lack of it, that Lee was receiving. I ended up writing my own IEP for Lee and presented it at another scheduled meeting. Some of Lee's goals included using reciprocal speech and interacting appropriately with other classmates and teachers. Fortunately, Lee moved on to junior high the next year, but I feel he wasted a whole school year in that class.

Lee's middle school and high school years were spent with a devoted teacher, Sandy Christman. She had such hope for "her guys." We exchanged a notebook most days. Her notes told me what went on and what to work on for the next day or week. I made her aware of any problems at home. Her notes to me were a lifeline. I counted on reading them when Lee got home because I had no idea what he did for eight hours out of the day. She was always so positive in her remarks. She really did seem to see Lee from a different standpoint. To me it was like she had a window into his mind, understanding why he did the odd things that he did. I always appreciated her insight and her devotion to her students. My replies to our journal were the last thing I did before I collapsed into bed at night. She has stayed a lifetime friend.

Lee was fortunate to stay in the school system until the age of twenty-one. At age eighteen, he was enrolled in a prevocational program at the Berks Career and Technology Center where he learned basic assembly-line skills along with practical living skills. I was thankful for the caring teachers that Lee was afforded there. I was also very thankful Lee could gain more proficiency for what I hoped would be employment after his graduation.

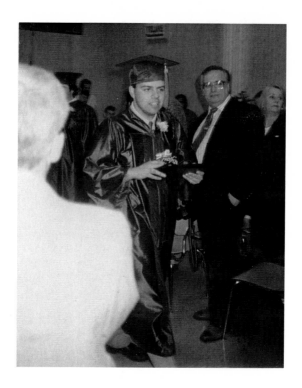

"Graduation Day!

Lee had one friend from high school that he still sees today through various programs for the disabled. His friend, Neil greets him each and every time he sees him in the same way. Neil touches Lee's face and talks about Bugs Bunny. Lee allows him to do that with a smile on his face. This has been their trademark greeting to each other for so many years. Neil talked to Lee and Lee listened. They both appeared happy, and then they went their separate ways. Most people don't understand their friendship, but the important fact is that they have one and it has survived the test of time!

After all these years, Lee is still invited back to his alma mater at the end of May for a graduation celebration and dance for the recent graduates. It's a night he always looks forward to, as do so many other graduates of the program. It's like a homecoming. We usually get him a new pair of slacks and shirt for the occasion and we were sure to have him shaved with a new haircut and looking his best.

I always accompanied him to the dance and got him settled in, and then I would blend into the background and watch him handle himself to the best of his ability. He loved the music that the DJ played, all the fun songs that young people enjoy at parties. At those dances, I got to see first-hand that Lee had a soft spot for one particular girl. Lee knew Jenny Sue for several years at school. Under different circumstances, she could have been his high school sweetheart! He lit up whenever he saw her. He searched her out to sit with her. She would want to dance with him and he tried to dance, but was always distracted and then he would go to sit down and be content to watch her dance with her friends. He just didn't know what to do. Everyone from the school was so glad to see him those evenings and to hear from me about all his accomplishments the previous year.

When I look back over the years since Lee finished formal education, I am amazed at how we managed. The one thing that I found out is that if I wanted something to happen, then I had to take ownership of the situation and do it myself. Sure I had IEPs and Individual Support Plans (ISP), but for the most part, Lee was one of the many disabled people who had specific needs. There were only a few social workers willing to offer directions or suggestions for Lee's future, as their caseloads were filled with so many other people. The job ultimately was up to me.

CHAPTER 8:

RAYS OF HOPE

In treating any ailment, therapy to address the problem is key to recovery. Therapy provides structure, progress measurement, and rays of hope for those afflicted. With autism during the 1970s and 80s, many of the therapies were based on unproven assumptions and subsequent methods, for a condition that no one could seemingly understand. Regardless of the efficacy, I always tried to treat autism with a solid dose of these methods. As a result, Lee's life always had an undercurrent of one therapy or another. The names and structures of the treatments changed from year to year, but hope was the constant.

In the late 1970s, I was willing to do almost anything to help Lee. I was instructed by a therapist to visit the local adult entertainment store for a purchase for Lee's therapy. I never in my wildest dreams thought I would be directed to purchase a sex toy to use specifically on my child's arms and legs for tactile stimulation, but I did what the therapist told me to do.

With the boys in tow, I calmly asked the store clerk for a vibrator. She asked me what size. I thought for a moment.

John always stressed to me that we didn't have to buy the most expensive item nor the cheapest item in regards to appliances and household items, so I told her to bring me the medium-sized vibrator. I still had no idea what I was asking for. Being so naïve, I never knew that those things existed, but, lo and behold, she came out of the stock room with a medium-sized plastic item that appeared to be a penis! I still did not think anything of it. If a therapist told me to do something, by golly I was going to do it! I used that vibrator faithfully on Lee's arms and legs twice daily for several years. It sat in our therapy basket in our living room for the sole purpose of tactile stimulation for our autistic son. Eventually, I did purchase another vibrator that did not look like a penis. I guess I led a more sheltered life growing up in Shillington, Pennsylvania, then I realized, because it was only years later that I actually learned what that vibrator was intended to be used for. For the record, John never commented about it either, but I suspect that when Matt was a teen he might have wondered!

I was introduced to Dr. Delacato's philosophy by Carol, the mother of one of Lee's classmates. Carol was taking her son Danny to Dr. Delacato, and she felt he was helping her son cope with the outside world. Danny's language skills were much better than Lee's, so I hoped that Lee could benefit from this approach. I talked to John about the possibility of us taking Lee to the Chestnut Hill Reading Clinic. I knew it would be another financial burden on John, but he agreed and we moved forward. The Chestnut Hill Reading Clinic was a place where children diagnosed as autistic and brain damaged came from in and out of the state. Besides our own home, the only other places I felt safe and comfortable taking Lee with all of his different behaviors were to my parents' house, where he received unconditional love, and to Dr. Delacato's center in Plymouth Meeting, Pennsylvania.

When I met other parents in the community or at Matt's or Billy's school events, each encounter presented a painful rehashing to explain Lee's autism diagnosis, an intimate problem I still hadn't come to terms with. In fact, I lived in denial for many years that Lee was truly autistic.

Dr. Delacato offered a wonderful respite for weary parents of autistic children, a place of hope and promise as we struggled with helping these puzzling children. With Dr. Delacato, we learned how to use treatment concepts from a team of therapy providers. Each child was tested and observed by the team in order to find the area of their senses that was affected the most. The senses of smell, touch, hearing, and sight were distinguished for therapy. We drove more than an hour to these exciting appointments, but others came from much further away seeking help for their children.

Dr. Delacato also had several treatment centers throughout the world in places such as Italy, Spain, Germany, and Israel. He always had us believe that we could beat this thing called autism. He stressed how important family was in dealing with Lee and he explained how our family had an important role in Lee's outcome. The therapists made us truly believe we could turn Lee around.

Dr. Delacato took Matt and Billy aside and told them that someday Lee would not have the label of "autistic" behind his name. I still can see their eyes when the doctor told those two brothers that someday Lee wouldn't be autistic. The look was as if they were imagining how life could be without Lee having this problem. How much easier it would be if he were like other boys. Looking back on that day, to me it was a sense of false hope that was given to them. We all know now that autism isn't cured.

Back home, we faithfully did Lee's therapy for at least forty-five minutes to an hour, twice daily. The therapy consisted of rolling and spinning Lee and providing tactile stimulation by rubbing a piece of shag carpet on his arms and legs. We put him through exercises to work on dominant hand and eye coordination. We tried to stimulate what skills he might have missed as an infant. When Lee was an infant, he only commando crawled, never grasping the concept of getting on his hands and knees to move. Using this treatment approach, we tried to get Lee to crawl around the house. We worked on the skills they prescribed for three months, and then returned for a progress report and a new set of skills to apply. We faithfully did this for several years. It was quite expensive to take Lee to these appointments, but John worked very hard so that we could keep trying to increase Lee's chance of improvement.

The therapy gave us hope and purpose that we were helping our son. Looking back, I always expressed that there was not one specific thing that made a big difference for Lee, but each try at something new, I felt, would help form him and help eliminate his problem areas. Small tasks for big results, I envisioned.

In the 1990s, Facilitated Communication, initially developed in Syracuse, New York, was a new concept in communicating with the autistic population. There were news articles and television specials touting the success that autistic individuals were experiencing. If given the chance to type on a keyboard, they could communicate and respond to answers to specific questions

As the concept trickled down to Pennsylvania and Berks County, I was given a keyboard to try the therapy with Lee. I was very suspicious of this, because I truly felt that Lee didn't have the ability to form the language to either speak it or to type it. Of course, I tried it on him anyway. We worked several evenings sitting at the kitchen table. I asked him a specific question such as "Lee, what color is the sky?" His response would usually be, "Yes." I tried over and over again, calmly asking all sorts of questions. I didn't want Lee to feel any frustration from me. Other than the obvious answers that I knew he knew such as, "What is your name?" he was unable to answer other questions. I was discouraged, because I kept hearing about all of the people who were responding to this therapy. I tried and tried with him, but eventually gave the keyboard back to the school.

After several months, Facilitated Communication was back in the news again. This time it was being reported that the persons helping the autistic individuals on the keyboard were actually the persons answering the questions! It has since been found to be a scientifically discredited technique. I then felt relieved that it wasn't me, or the method of how I was trying to make it work for Lee. It just didn't work.

Sometimes therapy can be fun. It has been thought for years that music has a positive effect on those with autism. To explore this path, I contacted a wonderful person who has since become a cherished family friend. Cindy Long was a special education teacher at a local Catholic school. She was also a music therapist. She agreed to meet to try to teach us the art of guitar playing. I say, us, because I thought if I learned then I could also work with Lee and teach him as well. A funny thing happened in the process. Lee took to the guitar so much better than I did! Cindy was surprised at how easily he adapted to the instrument. His love of music and the repertoire of songs she had him play were very enjoyable to him. I didn't mind bowing out of this endeavor, as it was very clear to me that I didn't have the same ability as Lee. Quite simply, I couldn't keep up!

More than twenty years later, Lee still enjoyed his weekly guitar lessons with his good friend, Cindy. She came to the house faithfully each week to encourage Lee to use parts of his brain that didn't get used often during the rest of the week. When you think of the tasks: reading the music, locating the chords and frets, playing the instrument, and singing along are not very easy to do, honest! He is now very familiar with the music of Billy Joel, John Denver, Elton John, and Kenny Rogers. He also enjoys the songs from musicals, such as *Fiddler on the Roof* and *Annie*, to name a few. He can go through the music from our church hymnal as well as all the basic children's songs. He has a playlist of songs for each holiday. I am so very proud of his accomplishments.

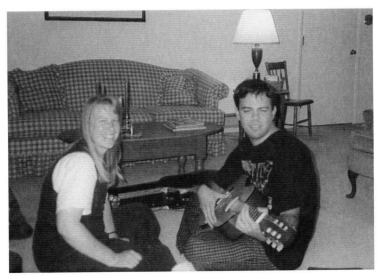

"Enjoying Guitar Lessons"

It was difficult for us to get Lee to play his guitar at other times, except for his weekly lesson. It was as though he didn't realize he could play for enjoyment and relaxation. He only knew to play it at his weekly lesson.

It would have been wonderful if he had played carols at our Christmas family gatherings or for his co-workers at his vocational workshop. I was very thankful that he played it when he did. I always made sure to be preparing dinner while he and Cindy had their lesson in the living room so that I could enjoy my private concert.

While Lee was in junior high school, he was introduced to Special Olympics. Established in the 1960s, people with intellectual and physical disabilities were given the chance to get involved in sports, showing their potential instead of dwelling on their afflictions. Eunice Kennedy Shriver, who was the sister of President John F. Kennedy, founded Special Olympics. She had a sister with an intellectual disability, so she understood the difficulty that people with mental weaknesses had in order to enjoy and compete in athletics.

As a way to drive motor skills, socialization, and competitive spirit, Lee participated in the yearly spring track and field days at school, and he also learned to bowl and swim. Mrs. Christman faithfully took him to the high school pool, along with the other students, and taught them to swim. They weekly went to a local bowling alley for practice in bowling. They also practiced running and throwing a ball during their gym classes. Lee was lucky enough to have a high school boy take him to the gym and practice basketball several times a week. I felt that he was getting needed exercise, making his body stronger and stronger.

After leaving the school system, Lee continued to participate in Special Olympics. Our yearly routine over many years had been that from September through November, Lee bowled on a Saturday afternoon and from January through May, he'd swim on Sundays. It was wonderful exercise for him and he got to be around other people with various disabilities who were also looking for entertainment. The exercise was as important as the circle of friends. The volunteers never criticized the athletes, they always showed them support and friendship. Lee didn't have friends that he engaged with there, but I know he appreciated the activities. They encouraged the athletes regardless of their ability.

While these practices kept Lee engaged and physically active, it also provided me with a chance to take some time for myself: a walk, a quick trip to the grocery store, or a jaunt to the local mall.

For a few years, Lee participated in the Pennsylvania State Special Olympics, which was held at Penn State University. Athletes from all over the state competed in many athletic events such as bowling, bocce, soccer, basketball, track and field, and swimming, to name a few. Local athletes boarded a bus the first week in June and stayed in the college dorms for several days. They competed in events and had lots of social activities. They had a chance to feel independent as they went through the cafeteria line to pick out their own food. It was so good to see Lee go away for a few days and try something different. We were thrilled to see him get off the bus when he got home with medals around his neck. It was a wonderful experience I am sure, for all of the athletes who attended.

As the years have gone by, Lee has competed in many athletic events and has accumulated more than sixty medals; gold, silver, and bronze. They hang proudly in his room.

Years later, his young nephews and niece always thought he was an Olympian. They were in awe of his medals. We never downplayed the importance of his activities and receiving his awards.

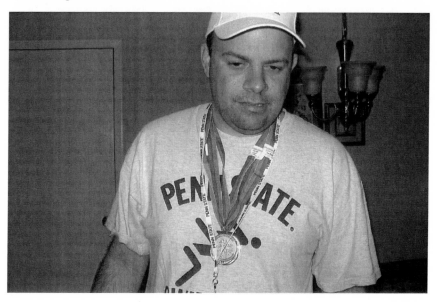

"Olympic champion and his Hardware"

CHAPTER 9:

GET TO WORK!

When Lee turned sixteen, I knew he had to start learning the concept of work. He had always been encouraged to produce in school, but the concept of getting up to go to work was not familiar to him. He did chores at home—taking out the trash, getting the mail, loading the wood box for our wood burner, and helping with gardening, but he did not truly know work.

There was a summer opportunity for underprivileged teens at Blue Marsh Lake, a recreation park near our home. I contacted the organizer and told him about Lee and his abilities. Lee was accepted into the program and hired to help clear the brush from the paths around the lake. Billy and I drove Lee to the spot near the lake where they were to begin their day's work, and we apprehensively drove away.

I waited nervously at home for the phone to ring. I didn't think Lee was prepared for the challenge, but felt he needed to start somewhere. It wasn't long before the phone rang and I was summoned to come pick Lee up immediately. I was told that Lee didn't understand what was expected of him. Apparently, he found it more appealing to throw stones into the water and watch the ripples form. Carelessly he put his shovel over his shoulder, unaware of the possibility of hitting another worker. I was told Lee should not return the next day.

We gathered up Lee and his belongings and drove home. Once again, in my safe place, I cried the whole way home, realizing how difficult the task of Lee at work was going to be. Billy once again tried to reassure me that things would work out and not to worry.

But I did worry. What was to become of this boy who was turning into a young man? What will his future be if he doesn't understand the concept of work ... a day's wage for a day's work?

I thought about the possibilities for him and wondered *what kind of work could he do? What were his strengths?* I knew he liked repetition and organization. My prayers were answered when Lee's aide at school had a contact at the local grocery store, who agreed to hire Lee for a part-time position in the bulk foods department. I volunteered my time to stay by his side and help him with quality control, making certain all packages were done as required. I was a job coach before they were in vogue.

Lee was shown his responsibilities and assigned two days a week to work, working three hours each day. The school district provided his transportation to the store after school, where I met him after my day's work was over. He bagged bulk food items such as licorice, raisins, noodles, and fig bars into one-pound bags. After placing the items in the bags, he weighed them, printed the labels, and then used a twist tie for closure. I watched him and assisted him if he was having any difficulty, making sure that his finished product was done correctly. I'd have to remind him to stay focused, to keep his hands away from his ears and not eat any of the products he worked with.

We were a good team, and he actually enjoyed his work bagging the items. He cautiously mastered the heat sealer, closing the bags without the twist tie. Lee's supervisor, who was a mother herself, realized that I had other family commitments at home, so she offered to take over the responsibility of checking his work. After I was no longer needed to help Lee, he was ready to work independently for a short period of time. We were very proud of him.

Lee remained at that grocery store for about two years. His job ended when new management, not receptive to people with disabilities, allowed co-workers to torment and ridicule him. I spoke to the store manager about his staff, but I felt the manager saw Lee as a burden to his store. He didn't have a problem with Lee's work; Lee just didn't fit in. Much of it was not apparent to Lee, but when Lee told me that he did not want to go to work, I realized he understood the cruelty of his coworkers. I knew it was time for him to move on. I didn't want him to work at the expense of his dignity. John and I could have filed a claim of unfair labor practices against the store, but we knew it would be exhausting work and that we had to keep focused on moving in a positive direction for Lee.

Before Lee graduated from high school at the age of twenty-one, he was fortunate to have had a volunteer position at Boscov's, a local department store, which later turned into a paying job. He worked in the sales-audit department, organizing the sales receipts from the cash registers from all of the branch stores. He sorted the receipt envelopes from each cash register in alphabetical and numerical order. He loved this work! He had a very supportive group of female co-workers who appreciated him tremendously. He worked rigorously to have all his work completed by the end of his work-day. His two-day-a-week employment at that store was a highlight of his life. He and our family felt like his co-workers were family.

Fittingly, those wonderful women of the sales audit department were recognized by the Pennsylvania Office of Vocational Rehabilitation for working with Lee the same year that Lee was recognized as Employee of the Year by the Office of Vocational Rehabilitation. We attended a banquet where he and the women were recognized.

We often treated his co-workers to sandwiches for lunch and found other ways to express our appreciation for their kindness to Lee. It's the least we could do! It was so apparent that his friends adored him. He was accepted into the fold of these charming ladies. When he acted out and had outbursts, they let him alone until he settled himself down. One of the women always took her lunch at the same time as Lee did to keep him company. I know it couldn't have been all fun working with Lee some of the days, but they never mentioned anything to me. Unlike his previous job, here he was treated with dignity and respect. They were angels.

The weeks leading up to Christmas were especially hectic in his department. Because of all the sales at all of the stores, Lee worked frantically to clear his space of envelopes before the end of his work-day.

Sadly, in February 2008, after sixteen years of employment, Lee was laid off from his job at Boscov's. The economic downturn at that time was very hard on businesses, and Boscov's management had to eliminate the positions of many full-time employees who supported families. I couldn't have expected them to keep Lee for his two-day-a-week position. I drove him home from his last day of work, knowing we just lost something very special. He has never again worked with such an amazing group of caring individuals.

Losing that job at Boscov's meant Lee had nothing to occupy his time during the day. I tried to keep him busy by having him do chores around the house, run errands with me, and do simple exercises. But I struggled with him not being productive with his time, knowing that when he went to his room, most of his time was occupied in repetitive behaviors such as listening to his John Denver cassette tapes over and over again, rewinding them to places where he enjoyed either the words or the music. He'd watch the same *Three Stooges* videos over and over, looking for the funny parts that made him laugh out loud. He'd always watch the clock or use his calculator. He never complained about spending time in his room; he actually loved it.

Once again, I was looking for another job for Lee. I convinced the manager of another grocery store to give him a chance to work a few days a week in the produce department, shelving produce such as apples, oranges, onions, and bananas. Though I never forgot about his past experience with co-workers who lacked compassion for the disabled, I thought it was an isolated incident. Unfortunately, however, I found out I was wrong.

Despite the Americans with Disabilities Act of 1990 requiring reasonable accommodations for the disabled, we once again found our son dealing with co-workers who could not find compassion to help him in the slightest way. Because of Lee's unusual behaviors, such as whining and holding his hands over his ears, the staff did not welcome him nor accept him. Lee got upset and had outbursts because of his frustration at not being able to communicate with them. I was called into his work on a few occasions to take him home. When I discussed with Lee the reasons he was sent home he listened, but he didn't understand the gravity of the situation. There were no guarantees that it wouldn't happen again. We could not predict what he would do or when he would do it. It was always the unknown.

Lee was afforded a job coach through an employment agency in coordination with the Office of Vocational Rehabilitation. This should have been enough for most people, but the coach showed Lee the requirements of his job and only stayed with him for a short time to get him settled in before he left Lee to work on his own. Lee needed more supervision initially, but those were the rules that we agreed upon.

What none of us realized was how alienated Lee was from the rest of the workers. Staff refused to work with us to help Lee find success. I often shopped in the store, and when I passed his co-workers they found it difficult to look me in the eye. I felt that they knew their behaviors were hurtful. We approached them cautiously over and over again to ask them to assist Lee in small ways, but we didn't want them to be angry with us and relay that anger to Lee.

The staff typically loaded the cart for him in the morning and then Lee was on his own to unload and shelve the produce by himself without any assistance. It's hard to imagine what it must have been like for him to again be working in a place where he wasn't wanted. He was the kid on the block who didn't have any friends. Leadership starts at the top, and when the management didn't enforce the love-thy-neighbor commandment, neither did the staff.

Lee worked two days a week at this store for a few years before being cut back to one day weekly. Perhaps they felt that cutting back his hours would make him quit. Monday mornings were dreaded. He would say to me, "Mom, no work." I told him he needed to work. Everyone needs to work at something.

Trying to seek employment for Lee, I later realized that this job wasn't benefitting him. In order for people with autism to be successful at their jobs, they need to have a good support system around them. I was told that the store management was getting complaints from customers because of Lee's detachment and his inability to answer their questions. When Lee was unsure of a situation, he held his hands at his ears and talked to himself, and these peculiar behaviors were alarming to customers. Lee's co-workers could have helped him by intervening on his behalf.

It was a snowy, icy Martin Luther King Day when an incident occurred that made me realize Lee needed to leave the toxic environment where he worked. He was scheduled to work his shift from 9:00 a.m. to 3:30 p.m. that day, just like any other Monday. And just like any other Monday, I thought his companion, Felix, was scheduled to pick him up at the end of his shift to take him out for an afternoon and evening of fun.

Companion services were intended to get disabled individuals into the community and learn skills necessary for independent living that would hopefully be useful in the future. Felix was a very caring and compassionate man who was very reliable and Lee looked forward to his outings with him. They always went out to dinner and then to the mall. Lee enjoyed going to the arcade and visiting the music stores where they looked for old tapes of Lee's favorite artists

About 7:30 that evening the temperature dropped below freezing and our roads began to get icy. I called Felix to warn him about the roads and suggested he should start heading home. To my surprise, Felix told me that Lee was not with him. Unfortunately, Felix forgot to tell me that the agency that employed him was closed on Martin Luther King Day. He assumed I knew he was off of work for that day. It was a terrible miscommunication.

What? Where was Lee? I panicked. This was four hours from the time Lee was dismissed from work, and where could he be if not with Felix? I quickly called the store to ask them to check to see if Lee might be standing outside the store waiting. The young lady who answered my call seemed to be annoyed with my questions and concerns. She went to look for Lee and later came to the phone to say, "Yes, he's out there." I quickly responded, "Please go get him into the building and buy him something to eat. He has money in his wallet. I will be right there to pick him up!"

As panic settled in, the tears started to flow. John and I quickly got into the car to head the seven miles to the store. *How could they not notice him standing there for more than four hours? Was he invisible? Why didn't someone ask about the guy standing out in the cold for so long? How could they be so uncaring?* We raced into the store to find Lee sitting on the bench inside with a look of abandonment on his face. His ears were so red and his body was so cold from standing out in the frigid weather for so long. He didn't understand what had just happened. John asked the sales associates how they could not have seen him standing there for so many hours. They just brushed off the incident with annoyance at our dilemma. We got Lee into the car, went through a drive-thru to get him some food, and drove him home. He immediately took a hot shower and then quickly went to bed. I went in to talk to him before he fell asleep, trying to explain to him what had happened and that he is safe and sound now. His only comment to me was, "Thanks, Mom."

How long could he have stayed out there in the freezing weather? When would someone have realized that he needed assistance? How many shoppers went inside to purchase their groceries and came back outside to see this young man still standing in the cold? Four hours of waiting and waiting. Was there not one compassionate person who passed by him that would have noticed he was in distress?

This incident was the last straw, and I knew Lee had to quit working at such an uncaring place. I realized how open Lee was to being taken advantage of. I have always been his protector for so many years, but when a caring adult is not around him, anything could happen. Thankfully, nothing harmful happened to Lee this time. *Thank you Lord.*

CHAPTER 10:
DEAR GOD, HOW MUCH CAN WE TAKE?

When Lee was twenty years old, in the wee hours of the morning in May of 1993, I heard what I thought were animal sounds from outside. It was warm and I had the windows open for fresh air. As I tried to sleep, I still heard this sound and then realized it was coming from the bedroom that Lee and Billy shared. Matt was in college at the time, and John had already left for work. I rushed into the room, turned on the light, and saw Billy standing over Lee.

Billy said, "Mom, there's something wrong with Lee!" As I got to Lee, I could see he was dazed and unaware of what was happening. I instructed Billy to call 911.

This was before GPS navigation systems were available. As Billy sat in the chair, his face pale and horrified, he tried to direct the ambulance driver to our house. The ambulance personnel were not familiar with our rural location. I will never forget the look on Billy's young face as he tried to direct the ambulance to our house without success. At that point, I realized it was up to me to get Lee the help he needed, so we managed to get him into the car and sped to the hospital which was thirty minutes away. We could see that he was breathing okay, but we knew something was terribly wrong with him. Our drive seemed to take forever till we arrived at the hospital.

Upon arrival, Lee seemed to have somewhat recovered from the episode. Billy and I looked at each other in disbelief. *Did this really happen? Should we be here?* I thought. I expressed to the intake nurse that I wasn't sure what had happened, as Lee seemed to be much more responsive than earlier. She looked at Lee and saw the bite marks on his tongue, and realized he had a seizure. She nodded and said, "Yes, it is good you are here."

Lee was examined and taken to another room for a CT scan. I accompanied him to the x-ray room, but was not allowed to go in with him for the test. Lee was unsure about what was happening to him, and I was unable to reassure him that it would be okay. After a few minutes, they wheeled him back out and we waited for the results. A group of doctors read the results, and one of the doctors informed me that it appeared Lee had a brain tumor and we should contact our family doctor.

How could this be happening to Lee? That was the question that went through my mind over and over again, *please God don't let this happen to Lee!* I immediately took him to Dr. Shippen for an examination, where I thought I'd be reassured that everything would be okay. When Dr. Shippen read the CT scan results, he immediately referred us to a local neurosurgeon that he respected.

We were able to schedule an immediate appointment with a neurosurgeon named Dr. Johnson, who ordered a Magnetic Resonance Image (MRI) of Lee's brain. I had no idea what an MRI entailed, but I knew it would be traumatic for Lee. He was given medication to calm him so he would remain still for the test. I accompanied him into the room and stood at his feet as they placed a helmet over his head and aligned it properly in the machine. Lee was told not to move, but I knew he didn't understand the gravity of their orders. The sounds of the MRI machine were deafening to me, and to this day I do not understand how Lee was able to successfully complete the test.

A few days after his test, we had an appointment with the doctor for a consultation. The doctor informed us that Lee did indeed have a brain tumor located in the left temporal section of his brain. Since Lee had autism, the doctor was very cautious about recommending brain surgery for him. We were told to wait six weeks to see if the tumor would grow. Those six weeks were so difficult for our family. Lee was unaware of his situation and continued to live life normally. I, on the other hand, was devastated. *How could this be happening to Lee? Didn't he have enough to deal with in his life? How could this young man deal with yet another trauma?*

I didn't need another test to tell me that Lee's tumor was growing. He became more and more restless. All of his unusual behaviors became more pronounced. He was con-stantly talking to himself, pacing, holding his hands at his ears, and whining incessantly. There were times that I felt I couldn't breathe. I would go outside and walk around the yard during the evenings, feeling desperate and frightened. John felt helpless also. Matt and Billy reassured us that Lee would be okay. When I spoke to my mother, I could hear the sadness in her voice, but she always tried to sound hopeful. There was nothing we could do but wait.

At the time, I was working at the high school as a guidance resource aide. It was the middle of May, and I needed to work every day till the end of the school year in June. I was consumed with worry, but working with the students regarding their career choices, job opportunities, and community-service hours helped take my mind off my problems. Summer vacation finally arrived; I could be home, be myself, and deal with whatever was about to come my way. I would never give up trying to make life better for Lee, but this problem was definitely out of my control.

After the six weeks elapsed, Lee had his follow-up MRI. A few days later, Lee had his appointment with the Dr. Johnson. John had to work, so I took Lee to the appointment alone. With test results in hand, we stopped at my mother's house for support before his appointment. Holding the x-rays up to the light of my mother's kitchen window, I tried to convince myself that the tumor in the second MRI looked the same as the first and that everything was going to be okay. And then I prayed.

At the doctor's office, Dr. Johnson came into the room and read the x-rays. He studied the results closely and then read the radiologist's report out loud. "Appears to be a tumor, has increased in size and must be removed." *What? I could not believe what I was hearing.* I felt my body go limp; the only reason I was able to keep myself composed was because Lee was looking at me intently the whole time. He knew there was something going on, and he could tell by my body language that it was serious. He keenly kept his eyes on me as the doctor explained our next steps. Lee would be admitted to the hospital on July 6 and have brain surgery on July 7, 1993. I hid my tears and emotion so I could drive home safely without incident.

Everything after that day in the doctor's office was again like a bad dream. How could this young man, who was twenty years old, this autistic man who had so much to deal with in his life, be given the task of dealing with a brain tumor? How could I be the best mother for him and stay strong? I prayed and prayed, just as my mother told me over the years. I tried to be strong for my family but feared the worst.

Seventeen years almost to the day after Lee was first diagnosed with autism, we were dealing with another devastating diagnosis, a life-threatening diagnosis. The morning of July 6 was a very somber time for our family. Lee was actually going to the hospital to have brain surgery. Matt, home from college, was always good company for Billy. He was in charge of Billy for the day as we took Lee to the hospital.

When we arrived at the hospital, John and I took Lee to admissions and then accompanied him as he was taken to his room for preparation. It was arranged for me to also spend the night with Lee. All of these experiences were traumatic for him but he went with the flow the best way he knew how.

The night before surgery, there was a terrible lightning storm. It lit up Lee's room with flashing light. I trembled as I sat in the recliner, praying as hard as I could. *"Please Lord; give me strength to help my son get through this struggle. Please let Lee be okay."* It seemed to take forever for morning to come. I dreaded it but knew we had to face this straight on.

In the early morning light, Lee was wheeled away for surgery. John, Matt and I waited for updates as the surgery progressed. Thankfully, Billy had a traveling soccer game that weekend so he stayed with family friends. A family friend who worked in the hospital lab came and sat with us. She was so comforting and her presence made us feel so much better. Matt worked on his computer while John and I sat quietly, not able to concentrate on anything else but the seriousness of Lee's surgery. I kept praying and reminded myself of my mother's words to keep the faith...everything would be okay. Would it? How could our autistic son deal with the effects of brain surgery?

We finally got a phone call from the surgeon, who reported that Lee survived the surgery and the tumor was removed successfully. It was explained to us that the tumor was encapsulated so that they could sort of pluck it out of his brain. The tumor was a Level two cancerous glioma.

Lee was placed in intensive care. When John and I were finally allowed to see him in the evening, we couldn't believe our eyes. He was connected to so many tubes. His head was thickly wrapped with gauze and he was hooked to several monitors. I silently sobbed with pity for our precious son. He was sleeping peacefully, still sedated, not having any idea what was happening. We waited patiently for him to awake because we weren't sure what he was going to do when he realized he was confined to a bed and his movement would be limited. The nurses were also concerned about how he would handle the situation. When Lee awoke, his mind was foggy, but he was very calm. The medication sedated him and kept him from moving around in his bed. We comforted him the best way we could and tried to hide our anxiety.

Before long, the tubes started to come out one by one. Because Lee had difficulty tolerating the restrictions of the Intensive Care Unit that limited his ability to get out of bed and walk around, he was almost immediately transferred to a private room down the hall.

Unbelievably, four days after brain surgery, with forty six staples in his head, Lee was discharged from the hospital. The doctor, who was amazed at his progress, said he never had a patient leave the hospital four days after brain surgery. We happily took him home to recuperate.

As in everything else, Lee does not think abstractly, there is only black and white. He didn't think about what was going to happen next. He was in the here and now. This enabled him to deal with the situation and not think about the possible outcomes. He never thought about the possibility of dying. He didn't understand the gravity of brain surgery. He didn't think that this surgery could impact the rest of his life. He only knew the present.

He was indifferent to all the attention he was getting. Get well cards started coming in as did small gifts from family and friends. His grandparents were so happy to come and visit. He didn't understand all the fuss. When his favorite person, my mother, came to visit again the next day, Lee wanted to please her. In the past, he always did forward rolls for her. It was fun for him. So as in the past, he motioned that he would do a forward roll for her again. "No, no, no!" we screamed, catching him before he got down on the floor to perform for us. Needless to say, we have never encouraged him to tumble again.

On our follow-up visit with Dr. Johnson, he reiterated what he had said at Lee's discharge. He successfully removed the glioma which was a level two cancerous tumor. He told us that he removed it in its entirety and that he was not recommending radiation treatments for Lee because the radiation treatments might cause more problems for Lee. Dr. Johnson has reminded me over the years that Lee's tumor could come back and resurface in another area of his brain or body. Lee has had subsequent MRIs over the last twenty eight years and has been cancer free. *Thank you Lord!*

I silently hoped that Lee's autism would disappear after his surgery. I thought that maybe the brain tumor was causing some of Lee's problems. After many weeks of waiting to see changes, I realized that Lee's autism was not going to be cured by removing his tumor.

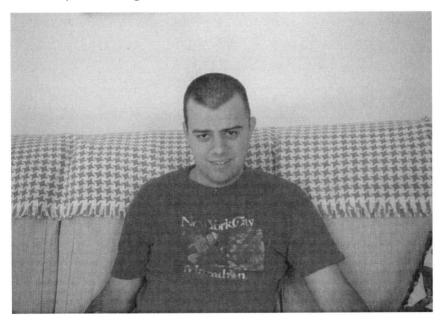

"Recovering from Brain Surgery"

CHAPTER 11:

COPING THROUGH WORK, MILES, AND FRIENDSHIPS

When Billy entered kindergarten, John and I decided that I should find employment in order to help with the bills and to start saving money for our boys' college educations. The only place I could consider was working for our local school district. Since I needed to be available to the boys when they were not in school, I initially took a substitute position working in the school cafeteria, easing myself into the day-to-day routine of being a working mother. I later secured a permanent position as a classroom aide, and a few years after that was fortunate to obtain a position in the high school counseling office. It was a full-time position during the school year and allowed me to have holidays and summers off with the boys. I was still able to schedule appointments for the boys for after school or during the summer, and it allowed me to contribute financially to the family.

My employment at the high school was a godsend; I met the most wonderful people there and I found joy in helping the students. I was able to leave my problems at home and deal with them at the end of the work-day.

Finding time to do Lee's tactile therapy, get house-work accomplished, plan meals to meet Lee's needs, and take care of the rest of my family was a lot to have on my plate, but I felt up to the challenge. Sometimes I look back and wonder how I did it. The days were very long, and I usually got about five hours of sleep nightly. My days were filled with attending after-school sports and activities and giving all of the boys the attention they so greatly deserved. Matt and Billy were very good boys, rarely giving me reason to discipline them. They did well in school, which allowed me to give more attention to Lee and his needs.

Through the years, I always said that Lee was fortunate to have a big brother who pulled him from the front and a little brother who pushed him from behind. That is still true! The love and support from these two guys who rose to the occasion every time in support of me from the time Lee was a small child to dealing with all the decisions that are made for Lee's benefit now as an adult are impossible to name. Every time I needed or still need a question answered or a shoulder to cry on, I can call either one of them. They both have an incredible sense of humor, which is definitely a trait from their Pop-Pop!

When navigating through business-like questions, I contact one or the other or both. When we have meetings for Lee's future, they are always there. I feel so very secure in knowing that they have always been there for their brother after all these years. They have so many responsibilities of their own with their families and their work, but they always have time for me. They have taken over what John is not comfortable helping me with … advocating for Lee.

The days, weeks, months, and years went by so quickly. It was not too often that John was able to help with the daily routine of working with Lee. I always felt his emotional support and his ability to provide for us financially enabled us to pursue expensive tests and appointments with specialists who we hoped could help us with Lee's autism.

When I reminisce about how I as a mother coped with Lee's disability, I think of all the support I received from John. He always provided silent support that demonstrated his concern for Lee and his appreciation for my initiative on Lee's behalf. He was coping the best way he knew. We are two entirely different personalities, both hurting in the same way. He was not a talkative man; he was a thinker, a person who stood back and analyzed the situation. He didn't always have suggestions of what to do to help Lee, but he always supported me in whatever choices I made. Whether it was Lee's daily therapy that we did twice a day, the various doctor appointments, or the all-natural diet that I produced for Lee, I always felt John's silent support. I knew that I wasn't alone in this.

In the summer months for many years, John umpired local softball games. This was money that he put aside for us to go on summer vacations to our beloved city of Cape May, New Jersey. This was also one way that he coped with the stress and demands that his family placed on him. We often packed up the boys and went along with him to the games because the games were often located near playgrounds. It was a wonderful release for the boys and it gave me a chance to talk to other women who accompanied their husbands who were playing on the teams. I often got glances and stares from some of the people because of Lee's unusual behaviors. We always made light of it, but deep down it hurt me terribly.

During their teenage years, Matt and Billy became very helpful with household chores. It was not uncommon for Matt to do the laundry, some food prep, and the yard work. When he was a young child, and I was pregnant with Billy and unsure of my life's situation, I heard Matt in the bedroom with Lee, helping him put the buttons in the box. "Lee, put the button in the box," Matt said, emphasizing the "b" sounds. I cried when I heard how he was trying to help his little brother understand many confusing concepts of the English language. His help continued throughout the years, and now, as a grown man, when I am struggling with various problems in regards to Lee, I can count on his insight.

Billy had his unique way of understanding Lee and finding the silver lining of every awkward situation he presented. He had many friends he brought to the house, and he was always comfortable with Lee and Lee's behaviors. His friends, one of whom ended up being his wife, always treated Lee in such a normal, caring way. There is never a time, to this day, that when I call him on the phone or text him a message that he doesn't reply almost immediately.

After Billy graduated from college and got a job that included travel, he actually took Lee to Disney World for a vacation. He could have taken anybody, but he chose Lee! He had a four-day conference to attend, and Lee hung out with him as his guest! The pictures and the stories of their vacation were hysterical. Lee had a ball, and I'm sure it was a moment to remember.

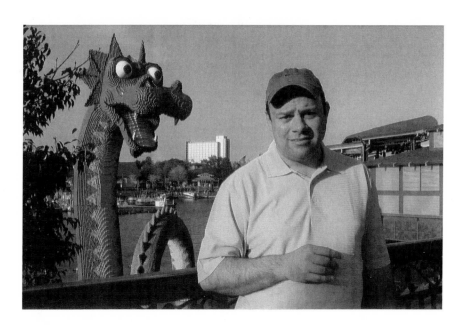

"Enjoying the Happiest Place on Earth"

My parents were unbelievably supportive with whatever I did for the children. They transported Lee to several of his appointments, especially his weekly visits to Easter Seals. Lee went to Easter Seals until he was seventeen years old. That's a long time to be a chauffeur! They always were my salvation when one of the boys was too sick for school. I could count on my parents to stay with the boys so that I could go to work.

My parents brought dinner from a local fast-food eatery to my house every Wednesday. After dinner John, who took on the position of treasurer of his union, left to work on the books. My dad and I went to the grocery store, and my mother stayed with the boys, giving them a chance to work on homework and have play-time.

I always kept my Saturdays for my mother. I loaded the boys in the car and we went shopping and out to lunch or we stayed at her house for the boys to play. As the boys grew,

Matt and Billy had other things to do with their friends, but Lee and I always seemed to end up at Nana's house. We continued our weekly rituals until my mother was too old and frail to do it any longer. Then we visited her in her nursing home and reminisced about the years gone by.

Later in life, the weekends that Lee and I spent together were just extensions of our trips to Nana's house years earlier. I always kept part of my Saturdays for his enjoyment. It became a bit of a juggling act when grandchildren came into the picture and I wanted to attend their events, so I had to be creative. Lee didn't care when or how he got to his destinations, as long as he got to go somewhere and get a special treat. If I bought him ice cream and we went into at least one store, he was very happy. He was and still is very easy to please. We tried to vary his entertainment, but as soon as we got home, he enjoyed himself once again with his cassette tapes, videos, and calculator.

Through the years, I always needed to have a project to work on to help take my mind off of my challenges with Lee. This enabled me to escape into a craft or to sew clothing for myself. I found joy in making curtains or a quilt for the house. When I had extra time, I would paint a room or even clean! I had to have something to think about other than my problems. I would let the thoughts come into my mind, but then I would release them again. To this day, I enjoy nothing better than making a Halloween costume for one of the grandchildren, decorating a birthday cake, or making a pot of soup. Staying busy was always my escape.

After noticing the relief I received from running, John, who was struggling with extra weight and the responsibilities of our family, decided to take up the hobby as well. He started out running to the mailbox and then down the road a bit, going farther and farther each week. Before we knew it, we were running two, four, and six miles a day!

We entered local road runs, taking turns watching the boys. Sometimes, when Matt got older, we had him watch Lee and Billy so we could run together in the local road races. I knew Lee was probably not being constructive with his time when he was on his own. I figured he was throwing stones in the creeks nearby, watching the ripples form, mimicking a clock with his fingers, or possibly he was at the playground, looking at the angles of the equipment. I had to let it go and let him do what made him happy. I knew that we would be reminding him not to fixate on those things when I got back.

We met the nicest people at the races, people that have become life-long friends. These friends never questioned us about anything or anyone in our family. They knew we were dealing with a very difficult and confusing dilemma, so they made our time with them so enjoyable. We laughed, and loved all of the silliness they provided. Before long, John was running marathons and it became our family pastime to travel to different cities and towns for road runs. We picnicked and partied with all of the different families. We had a wonderful time, and it was just what our family needed to get us through the darkness of the unknown. Our running family helped us tremendously, and I will never forget them for their friendship.

While running a local race, I wound up on a pace with another woman my age, who became one of my dearest and closest friends. Phyllis had three little girls who were about the same ages as my three little boys. We ran the same pace and decided to meet each weekend for a long run. Since our family responsibilities were most important, we'd meet about six on Saturday mornings while our children were still sleeping. We'd run our course, take a breather when we were finished, and hurry home in time for breakfast. With few exceptions, we met for more than fifteen years, running, talking, laughing, crying, and getting support to tackle motherhood for the next week. We shared stories and frustrations. She listened to me and I listened to her. She never questioned me about Lee unless I offered. I tried to take that one hour a week and not think about how difficult my life was. We often joked that we were running to improve our health and someday, when we were old in the home, we'd wish our hearts would stop but, because we had run so many miles, our hearts would keep going and going. We laughed and laughed, never thinking that one of us would one day be diagnosed with the curse of ALS, Amyotrophic Lateral Sclerosis, known as Lou Gehrig's disease. Phyllis was a woman who always ate healthy, loved wine, and exercised every day. She was a nurse and had a genuine love for people. She truly was my best friend and confidant for so many years, one I truly miss.

It was when Billy entered preschool that I met my good friend Nancy, who also has a great sense of humor. We hit it off from the start. Her son and Billy have the same birthday, and they were friends throughout school. Through the years, when I was struggling or if I had good news to share, I'd often call her and, before too long, we were laughing or crying about something. I always felt better after our conversations. It has helped me tremendously over the years to have her shoulder to lean on. Our friendship is about forty years old now and, unlike us, it hasn't grown old!

In my early days of retirement, and after Lee turned thirty-five, John and I were afforded some help through government services for Lee. Until that point, all of the treatments and programs for Lee were funded by our family. Social Services was finally addressing those with autism, and they began including them in the benefits which were traditionally provided to the more well-known and defined diagnoses like Down syndrome, physical disabilities, and others. Based on this support, Lee was able to engage with a number of companions who took him out socially and helped him to interact with a different dimension of the world than I could provide. They went to dinner, bowling, or to the mall, working on skills that would help him later in life.

Occasionally, they went for a hike or for groceries. Lee started to learn how to use the Internet on their visits to the library. John and I were then able to go out for dinner or just relax at home. It was definitely a help having someone else take over many of the social activities. I realized then that I was getting tired. Being Lee's social coordinator for so many years, I was ready to hand that part of caregiving over to someone else.

They say "it takes a village to raise a child," and I wholeheartedly feel this is true. I do not know how I could have survived those years without the love and support of my family and friends, and now the help of the state and Federal programs. The challenge is that you can't pick the size of your own village. It is interesting that some family members never called. I always thought it was because they didn't know what to say and felt so unsure of how they could help. As I look back, I'd say it was as though our village had a plague. That plague was called autism, and we dealt with it as well as we could with as many solutions as we could muster.

When I hear of children being diagnosed with autism, my heart sinks and then it goes out to the parents, the mothers especially, as this is a disability—like so many others—that will not go away with time. It's a lifelong disability that you can either shy away from or tackle head on for many, many years to come. I realize, however, that current treatments for autism are very different than what was available to Lee so many years ago. It is a much more hopeful disability than when Lee was diagnosed, and I thank God for the progress to help all those affected.

CHAPTER 12:
A SQUARE PEG IN A WORLD OF ROUND HOLES

Throughout Lee's life, we have never been at a loss for examples of how he does not recognize nor appreciate the abstract and the obscure norms of society and the implied danger in various life situations. This is true today, has been underscored countless times throughout the years, and was punctuated for all of us early in his life by an incident we had in the beginning of one summer.

The ocean has always been very soothing to Lee. As a very young child, he enjoyed the predictable rhythm of the waves crashing in. I often wondered what was going on inside his head. *Was it like a song for him, or did he count the seconds until the next wave arrived?* When he was older, he would stand in the water for hours with his hands at his ears and a smile on his face. Lee's uniqueness often drew stares from unknowing beachgoers. As we usually went to the same beach each day of our vacations, I was mindful to always sit near the lifeguards, and the lifeguards became familiar with Lee from year to year.

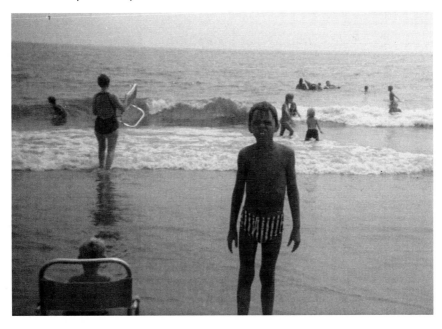

"Beach Bum..."

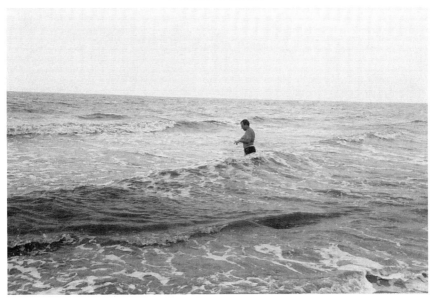

"...who was always in the water"

As John and I ran road races, we traveled to other cities and used these trips as opportunities to enjoy small vacations with our family. One of these races was held at the beach. After running the race, it was tradition to have a picnic, which included plenty of food and drink, with several of the other runners. It was an early-summer race, and the lifeguards were not yet on duty.

As we put our beach chairs down to relax, the boys immediately ran to the water. At the time, Matt was a teenager, Lee was twelve, and Billy was eight. As I diligently watched the boys play in the water, one of our friends came to talk to me and blocked my view of the boys. After what only seemed like a minute, and it might well have only been a minute, I looked with horror to see Lee and Billy caught in a riptide and unable to get to shore. As I screamed for help, several good Samaritans ran into the ocean with us to try to get them back to shore. It's all a blur as to who got which child, but they were brought to shore safely with our family's gratitude. The look of terror on Billy's and Lee's faces will be forever ingrained in my memory.

I realized afterward that I let someone interfere with my priority of taking care of my children, and I could have easily lost two of them that day. While Billy knew inherently what had happened and realized the mistake, Lee needed to have the black and white of the situation to understand and change his behavior. From that day on, Lee lines himself up with me on the beach. He keenly gauges where he should be in the water and how far out he should go by my hand gestures to him. He now has defined the risk and has a strict set of rules he follows to make sure it doesn't happen again. Since that incident, we have not had another similar encounter with the ocean; we are very careful and understand its might.

Typically, as people go through life, they learn life lessons and are able to transfer that knowledge to other situations and conceptualize the outcome. For Lee, generalizing is a concept that is very difficult for him to understand. He can be shown something that he should remember or apply to another situation, but this transaction in the brain is very difficult for him. As when he was waiting outside after work that snowy winter's night, we cannot expect he will be able to apply what he has learned to another situation. It forces me to always assume that Lee does not understand what is obvious to many of us.

Shortly after the beach incident, we were again reminded of Lee's lack of ability to think abstractly and the difficulty he had with generalizing. Living on two acres of land in a rural, wooded area, we enjoyed a lot of privacy. When the boys were busy playing outside, many times they didn't want to interrupt their play to come inside to use the bathroom, so they would just pee behind a tree or a bush.

On our family trip to Disney World when Lee was twelve years old, we enjoyed several trips to a water park known as River Country. The slides and water rides were so much fun for the boys. Matt enjoyed the big slides, while Lee and Billy were content to stay on the smaller ones. I could let my guard down because I felt we were not scrutinized and could do our thing without eyes watching us. I didn't have to explain why my little boy was intently watching the bubbles come out of the pool to the point of obsession or why he repeated a particular movement over and over again. Everyone was playing and having a good time when Lee urinated on the bushes next to the play area! We quickly reminded him that he couldn't do that in public and worked on that concept when we got home from vacation. Needless to say, no longer was it an option to pee behind the bushes at home.

Lee's concrete world has always revolved around structure, consistency, and rituals. A perfect example of that rigidity was in his multiple daily rituals, commitment to detail, and routines at home. Even if he awoke at four a.m., he stayed in bed until the clock displayed 6:15. He showered and dressed at the same time each day before he methodically took all of the laundry from the previous day downstairs. In the process, he stopped to take the previous day's newspaper to the basement to recycle. It didn't matter to him that we might not have read the paper yet. If we wanted it, it was filed in the recycling pile, always in order by sections.

As I noticed these habits and rituals, I began to see how Lee might be able to move to more supported independence. His work ethic, his determination, his commitment to finish what he began, and his accountability for what he did were similar to the traits that Matt and Billy possessed, though their work ethic was on a much higher level than Lee's.

Because of Lee's obsessive-compulsive behavior, he is meticulous about his surroundings and his bedroom is immaculate by his standards. There is not one item out of place. All of his CDs, DVDs, and books have a permanent place. If he uses something, it goes back to the exact spot where it came from when he is finished with it. He wouldn't notice if the dust were an inch thick, but he would notice if a CD was misplaced.

Lee knows only one speed. He does not understand what it means to hurry to accomplish a task. He never skips a step in completing a task, either. When we plan an event or a trip to shop, we are sure to give Lee plenty of time to tend to all of his habits so that we can leave on time. His clocks have to be synchronized and everything he used must be placed back in its appropriate position.

His nighttime rituals relied on structure as well. He woke up several times a night for so many years. He'd check the clocks in the house to see that they were all functioning properly, close cabinet doors that might be ajar, empty trash cans, organize newspapers in the basket by sections, open and close bedroom doors to check to see if everyone was sleeping, and open the refrigerator to inspect his packed lunch for the next work day. It was almost as if he had to do these tasks and check them off in his head. He had been doing this routine for so long that it became normal.

The whole time he was doing these things, he was talking to himself. Of course, he wasn't the only one whose sleep was interrupted. John sometimes heard him, but I always heard him. I understood how the lack of sleep could affect his health, but it was so difficult to tell him to stay in bed and not get up. Unable to find a solution, it just became our way of life. It didn't matter what medicine we gave him to calm him down during the day, he always woke up during the night to do his nighttime chores.

From a social and physical perspective, Lee was often distracted by pretty girls or, at his current age, pretty women. He has never had an encounter with another female. If we were at a social event and I was talking to another woman, Lee would interrupt and ask, "What is your name?" After the response, he would walk away and allow us to talk again.

I mentioned previously his soulmate, Jenny Sue. She is the exception to the rule. Lee has known Jenny Sue for more than twenty-five years, and I think of her as the love of Lee's life. He absolutely lights up when he sees her, and she's the only girl that he approaches independently. They smile to each other, he will ask her what she is doing, and then he walks away. It's sad that Lee cannot continue into conversation, and I often wonder how he feels. *Does he realize that he can't do what most of us can? In his mind, is his conversation complete?* He never looks disappointed to me.

Looking back at this lack of conceptual balance, I am struck by how difficult it must have been for him to process individual items. His horseback riding therapy is a memorable example. When Lee was young, we learned that children with various disabilities could benefit from horseback riding. Being able to feel the soothing rhythm of the horse was thought to help improve the child's muscle tone and body strength. Lee was also taught how to groom and clean up after the horses. As he went through the exercises of brushing their manes and coats, it was obvious by the look on his face how much he disliked the tasks. While he struggled to cooperate with the therapist, he made every effort to do as they said.

Imagine Lee being introduced to a horse named Squirrel at the same time we were trying to teach him what a real squirrel was. This was also true for Snowflake, a beautiful white horse that he rode. Oh, if he just would have gotten to ride Mister Ed, the talking horse from the 1960s sitcom. Often when we're out with the family, one of us will say, "Walk on," in reference to what Lee was supposed to say to his horses, Squirrel and Snowflake, reminiscing with a smile about Lee's horse-back-riding days.

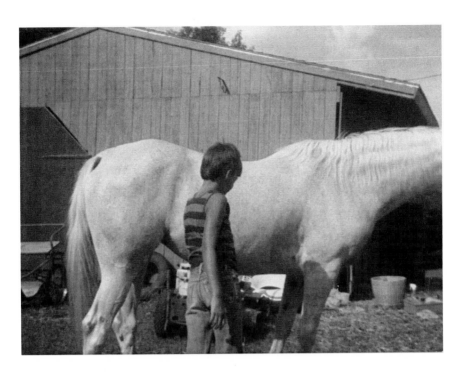

"Grooming his steed Snowflake"

Reminders that Lee lacked abstract thinking continued well into his adult life. When Lee was in his thirties and worked at Boscov's, the company always treated its employees to an end-of-summer picnic day at Dorney Park Amusements. It was held in September after the summer crowds died down a bit. There were two parts to the park, the amusement park rides and the water rides. Lee loved them all! The higher and faster a roller coaster went, the better he liked it. Unfortunately, I didn't feel the same way. I usually dreaded that day. I looked forward to Lee's enjoyment, but I knew I'd have to dig deep for the courage to go on all the rides with him. Kiddingly, I would ask myself why he just wouldn't be happy with the merry-go-round or the sailboats! As the roller coaster climbed to the top of the highest hill, he would look at me with the biggest smile on his face and say, "Thanks, Mom!" I'd respond jokingly with my standard reply, "The things I do for you, Lee."

When we got to the section of the park with the water slides, we had to change into our swimsuits. Since Lee was an adult, he had to change in the men's locker room and couldn't come with me to the women's locker room. We went our separate ways and I changed as quickly as possible so that I would be ready when Lee came out of his changing area. As I waited for him along the wall, he came out of the locker room bare-ass naked, asking me to get the knot out of his swim trunks! *What?* "Oh Lee, get back in there!" I exclaimed. I hurried him past all the stares from men, women, and yes, children, into the ladies room to change. Having no knowledge of how his behavior affected other people, he was not at all embarrassed and he had no clue how mortified I was for him at the time. I was so disappointed that he didn't understand how socially wrong that event was. I have since adapted to so many difficult situations over the years that, as I look back at that day at the park, I think, *who cares?* To this day, Lee can still walk through a room filled with people, wearing only his underwear, and not feel the least bit underdressed!

After that story, it's obvious that Lee doesn't notice his own appearance and we always seemed to think that, for the most part, he didn't notice our appearances either. But this theory was disproven one beautiful sunny afternoon at my niece's outdoor spring wedding reception. As the sun was shining through the tent that was set up for the occasion, my mother and I sat across the room from Lee. Sitting on the other side of the dance floor, he noticed a stray hair coming out of his grandmother's chin. He got up from his seat, walked intently across the dance floor to where we were sitting, and plucked that hair right out of her chin! *How did he see that? And how did he do that?* I was sitting next to my mother and I never noticed it! Unable to compose ourselves, we laughed and laughed. We reminisced about that day for years to follow.

CHAPTER 13:

YIELD TO A HIGHER POWER

Through the years, I've often felt very alone in my quest to find help for my son. I had family who cared, but ultimately it was up to me to solve the problem. With a sick feeling down in my gut, I wondered if there would ever be a breakthrough for him.

The specialists told me that his disability was incurable, but I remained hopeful when I heard of miraculous turn-arounds in several children, and I always remained prayerful. If I didn't have my faith, I don't know what I would have done.

While faith has always been an integral part of my life, it was my mother who encouraged me to take Lee to heal-ing services back in the 1980s. It was the rage at the time, and I was willing to try anything. *What harm could be done in taking Lee to church?* I reasoned. Several local Catholic churches held faith-healing services where a person who sup-posedly had divine powers laid hands on people who had varying degrees of illness. Sometimes my mother and I would witness the afflicted person actually pass out! I was sure that person would then be healed, though I never had any proof to support my conclusion.

When I took Lee up to the altar, the faith healer laid his hands on Lee's head and prayed for his healing. My mother and I were certain that Lee improved after being singled out and blessed. No one in the family challenged our beliefs; they just quietly allowed time to go by. I stopped going to those healing services when I recognized one of the healers at a local church. I found it questionable that she had healing and spiritual powers. At that point, feeling somewhat the duped victim, I had to admit that Lee really hadn't improved from these services. It was another example of trying anything to help him.

For several years, when Lee was a small boy and went grocery shopping with me, he would pick up an orange or grapefruit when passing through the produce department and hold it up in front of the mirrors that were located above the shelves. He would present it as though he was the priest and it was a communion wafer. Matt and Billy hid their laughter when they watched him, and it made me smile as well. My mother always thought Lee would one day become a priest!

As a grown man, Lee still follows the Mass closely, and church is very important to him. In his missal, he follows with enthusiasm all of the prayers and blessings that the priest says. He is clearly tuned in to what is being said and his mind never seems to wander, except during the homilies. He struggles to comprehend what the priest is talking about; quite honestly, sometimes I do too!

When Lee was in his early forties, our church offered a spirituality program that was led by a nun named Sister Mary, a woman with a beautiful heart. I was one of eight parishioners who took an oath of confidentiality and joined in the weekly discussion and prayer service. Participants could speak about anything that weighed heavily on their hearts, or they could choose to sit quietly without speaking. Every week I listened attentively to their stories and heard what they were dealing with in their lives. It was a very beautiful hour of peaceful prayer and reflection.

I attended these gatherings during a time when I was particularly struggling with Lee's future and what would happen to him when I was no longer able to care for him. Matt and Billy told John and me that we needed to think about placing Lee into another living situation. It weighed heavily on my heart, because I knew Lee was struggling with internal turmoil. He was very easily agitated and was unsettled in his behaviors. It was not uncommon for him to act out when he was unsure of what was happening. He reacted aggressively to loud voices and any type of confrontation. I couldn't possibly allow him to leave me and live with someone else when his behavior was so unresolved and volatile.

One week during the spirituality program, I found the courage to tearfully share my concerns about Lee with that small group of parishioners. Sister Mary suggested that I let it go to God. She reminded me that worry was not going to help the situation and that prayer would guide me down the right path. After a closing blessing, we headed to our cars in the parking lot.

Walking to my car, I physically felt a rush come across my shoulders and into my body. It lasted only a few seconds, but I truly believe it was the Holy Spirit letting me know that things would work out. I felt relieved and at peace as I drove home that night and didn't let worry about Lee's future overcome me again.

I shared my experience that night with only a few people, but I have never forgotten it. It was only a few short months after that incident that I was led to the answer for Lee.

CHAPTER 14:
LEE'S VERSION OF A CURE

Lee had the potential to be more independent and give more to society, but to be effective he had to get past all of the behaviors that held him back. His outbursts, anxiety, and holding his hands at his ears to avoid having to engage with others—all of these behaviors negatively affected his ability to live independently and find employment. I wanted him to snap out of it, but that just wasn't happening. For years, the medicines I gave him were only a temporary fix, and they often caused him to fall asleep. Lee required so much medicine to calm him down that it often seemed that we were drugging him in order to avoid his outbursts and inappropriate behaviors.

Dr. Shippen did a tremendous job helping Lee, both physically and mentally, and thanks to him Lee enjoyed excellent health. Anticipating Dr. Shippen's retirement in the not-so-distant future, I tried for several years to find a doctor to take his place. There had to be specialists who had additional information about medication benefits for the autistic population that could help Lee with the effects of his autism. There had to be someone who could give him the help he needed. We struggled to find a psychiatrist who would take him as a patient. Most times when I called a new doctor's office, the intake receptionist politely took our initial information and a few days later called back to say the doctor wasn't taking new patients at the time. This occurred over and over again. Lee was classified as disabled, receiving Medicare benefits and Medical Assistance because of his disability, and it seemed like the doctors didn't want to accept the lower payments that these entitlements reimbursed. Experts say that if someone needs mental health support it is available, but in my experience, I found that to be completely false. Perhaps it's true for a person who has the right insurance. However, a disabled person on a limited income requiring Medical Assistance might not be appealing to a doctor. My guess is that doctors were reluctant to see Lee because it was not financially beneficial for them to do so.

At Lee's annual follow up exam for his MRI, the physician assistant asked me if there was anything she could do for us. I asked her if she could recommend a doctor to treat Lee's autism. It happened that she did know someone who she thought would be willing to take Lee on as a patient. She gave me the contact information and I called that doctor's office the next day. I left Lee's initial insurance information, as I did with all the other doctors in the past, and a few days later I received a call from the secretary that this doctor would see Lee as a patient! I was elated! We scheduled our first appointment with Dr. Janiece Andrews, a psychiatrist in Camp Hill, Pennsylvania. Another prayer had been answered!

Lee and I drove to his appointment with Dr. Andrews on October 20, 2014. It was life changing for both Lee and me. Dr. Andrews and her staff greeted us warmly and made us feel very comfortable in her spacious office. She asked me to tell her about Lee and what I thought might help him. Trying to hold back my tears, I managed to get his history out, giving her a short synopsis of Lee's life. More than forty years of struggles in a few minutes is not an easy thing to convey. She was so calm and reassuring that I finally was able to get through telling his story.

I told her that I wasn't looking for a miracle cure, only a medicine that would help him cope with the commotion that was going on inside his body. I shared with her that I felt he was not on the proper medication for his disability, making it clear that I no longer wanted to over-medicate him for his anxiety and outbursts in order for him to cope with his world. I asked her if she felt she could help; she nodded and responded, "Yes." *Oh, my God. Could there be a medicine that would help him deal with day-to-day learning and living?* Before writing a prescription for Abilify, she had samples to offer us in order to find the level of therapy that Lee needed. I was instructed to observe him closely to see when or if the benefit of the medication would show. She gave me specific instructions and told me to contact her at any time if I had questions or concerns. We stayed in touch through phone conversations, making sure he wasn't taking too much or too little. She said I'd know when he was at the therapeutic level.

I was so excited to try this medicine for Lee that as soon as we got to our car, I gave him his first pill in the parking lot! I nervously glanced at him while we drove home, not knowing at all what I was looking for. Lee kept glancing back at me, probably wondering what all my excitement was about. I just hoped and prayed this was going to help him.

After a day, I noticed subtle changes in Lee's behavior. He seemed to quiet down, he held his hands at his ears less frequently, and he didn't chatter as much. I sensed he was acting calmer. He wasn't sleeping off medication as he had previously done. *Was I imagining it?*

The next day was noticeably better, and the following days were each better than the day before. He actually slept through the night for the first time in years. We no longer heard the sounds of cabinet doors slamming or waste cans being emptied in the middle of the night. Now Lee waited until the morning to check out his packed lunch in the refrigerator. Our bedroom door stayed closed. It was incredible!

It was obvious to me that Lee felt so much better, and John and I were thrilled by his progress! I received reports from his companions that Lee was so much easier to deal with on their outings. His supervisor at his workshop said Lee wasn't having outbursts any longer. He wasn't lashing out at me any longer, either. I was able to take him out in public and feel comfortable that he could handle himself appropriately.

The change in my son has been transforming. Lee had not known peace and serenity for so many years, and now he knows peace and serenity! I don't panic when I see new situations for him. And Lee has noticed the difference in himself, too! He is a different person. It is like night and day. He faithfully takes his medicine each day because he knows it makes him feel better. I am forever grateful!

Since that day in 2014, we routinely make our quarterly trip to Camp Hill to see Dr. Andrews. It's a fun day trip for us. We usually stop at Lee's favorite place for lunch and then get an ice cream cone at the dairy on the way home. It's a day I look forward to!

CHAPTER 15:

MOVING OUT

For ten years or more, I had been considering the options for Lee and his future living prospects. I knew that neither Matt nor Billy would be able to provide for him. I also knew that I would not want them to have to deal with Lee's daily living routine, and I certainly knew that my two wonderful daughters-in-law hadn't signed up for that when they said "I do." I weighed the possibilities of how long he could live at home with us.

One alternative living situation was Life Sharing, a living arrangement where a person with a disability chooses to live with a willing host family. It would be comparable to a foster home for the disabled, wherein the host family receives a monthly check to care for the individual. I was hesitant about this concept, because all families have flaws and imperfections. My imagination ran wild with the possible issues he could encounter, including people who lacked compassion.

Another possibility was a group home for people with disabilities. Caretakers at a group home give support to the disabled individual in all aspects of daily living by preparing their meals, laundering their clothing, providing companionship, and taking them to doctors' appointments. It is a home away from home. There were several homes in our area that offered this service. Though I didn't feel my requirements were unreasonable, it was difficult to find a place that offered everything I was looking for. For me, the hardest part was giving the responsibility of caring for my son to someone else. I loved everything about caring for Lee, and never saw it as a chore.

John and I were both getting older, but I was in good health and felt I could care for Lee for many more years. There was no way he could act out the way he did at home and be safely sent out into the world unless we could find an effective medication to control his outbursts. If this was my only option, I would keep him with me as long as possible and we would grow old together. I often saw elderly mothers taking their special loved ones to various activities and envisioned myself doing the same. *Did I have the courage to send Lee to live somewhere else? Could I find a place that was good enough for my son?*

When our immediate family got together for birthdays or holidays, I had to be aware of anything that would ignite the rage that was within Lee. When agitated, Lee made loud noises, grabbed our arms, and became aggressive. Matt and Billy often had to restrain him. At times, they even removed him from the house and took him for a car ride or a walk outside in order to calm him down.

When my grandchildren were around and something didn't go quite the way Lee thought it should, it sometimes set him afire and he would act as if he was going after one of the children. I usually babysat my grandchildren at their homes so as not to expose them to Lee's outbursts and to insure their safety, while John stayed at our house with Lee. We tried to figure out how to avoid things that triggered Lee, but it was normal family interactions that sometimes set him off. Lee just struggled to understand.

After Dr. Andrews placed Lee on the proper medication that enabled him to go through life in a calm fashion, our gatherings were pleasant and enjoyable. It took us some time to realize that this was our new normal with Lee. We no longer were afraid of what might happen. It was then that I felt comfortable revisiting the living situations that were available.

I considered the idea of respite care, which is exactly what it sounds like. It provides a place for the disabled to go for a day or a weekend while at the same time it gives the caregiver a rest. After researching this concept, however, I was not comfortable with the options and was concerned about the difficulties these situations could pose for Lee. The noise of a more urban setting when he was accustomed to the quiet of our rural setting, spending a weekend with people unfamiliar to him, and having Lee spend a weekend with people who were unfamiliar to me—all of these things made me apprehensive.

Our first step in making a transition started with Lee's guitar teacher. She was a trustworthy, caring person who was very comfortable around Lee. I asked her if she would consider coming to our home for a weekend so that John and I could get away for a few days and go to Cape May. Cindy agreed, and that was the beginning of our quest to find a place for Lee. After a few years of bimonthly visits to Cape May, I was more comfortable leaving Lee. He enjoyed his time with Cindy and his independence from me.

Lee had very dedicated paid companions who took him to all kinds of community activities. He also had habilitation workers who taught him how to navigate in the community. They reinforced his ability to order a meal at a restaurant, to give the right amount of money for a purchase, and to get the correct amount of change from a transaction. They even tried to teach him to do his own laundry. I saved Lee's laundry for a particular day and the habilitation worker would help him sort it and start the washer. After taking him out for dinner, they came back to the house to transfer the wash into the dryer. When time ran out, I completed the task. Lee worked with the habilitation workers on the chores they introduced to him, but at the end of the evening, he was very tired. He finished his work, got ready for bed, and was asleep in a flash.

I have always admired Lee. Many situations that most of us find quite simple were very difficult for him. He worked so hard to accomplish simple tasks and participate in social interactions.

Reacting to requests and prodding from Billy and Matt to help Lee take the next step, we visited several group homes in the area. I vividly recall the first home we visited on a cold Sunday in January following a snowfall. On this bleak day, as we entered the sparsely furnished living room, we were greeted by apprehensive group home workers who seemed uneasy with our presence. Absent were pictures on the walls, carpet on the floors, and that homey feeling. We were shown various bedrooms of the residents, some of whom were bedridden. *Could Lee fit into this kind of environment?* It didn't match my dream for him to find a bachelor pad where he could blossom and connect with residents with similar disabilities, a place he could call home.

After visiting several homes that accommodated residents with varying degrees of disabilities, I told Matt and Billy that those houses were not what I had in mind for Lee. They balked at my disapproval and tried to assure me that Lee didn't care if there were pictures on the walls or carpeting on the floors. They felt he didn't need anything special or homey, he just wanted to have his needs met. We certainly had our differing opinions and disagreements on what was appropriate for Lee. I told them I didn't want to consider the option any longer, and we didn't speak a word about that Sunday afternoon visit for almost two years. It was the proverbial elephant in the room whenever we talked about Lee's future.

How could this be so hard for me? Why couldn't I find a place for Lee that wouldn't compromise my values? I was adamant about finding a place that would not only be comfortable for Lee but would also make him happy, being fully aware that it was my duty and responsibility to make a suitable choice for Lee because he was not able to make the choice for himself.

In the fall of 2016, after Lee was on his medication and after careful consideration and many hours of prayer, I mentioned during Lee's annual Individual Support Plan (ISP) meeting that I would consider revisiting some homes for Lee. There was no hurry, as I envisioned us going into this slowly. Matt and Billy were taken aback because I had not mentioned anything about this to them earlier.

It became obvious to me that Lee was really getting bored living at home. He just wanted to spend time in his room, watching TV or listening to his favorite music. He came to dinner when I called, but he preferred to head back to his room after dinner. I also noticed that I wasn't able to keep up with the demands that this young guy needed. He is twenty-four years younger than me, and thirty years younger than John, and he wanted to do more than hang out with his aging parents! Both John and I were slowing down. It was time for Lee to leave the nest, and I needed to do the right thing for him.

Again, our family talked briefly about Life Sharing, but I truly didn't feel the connection with it. We talked about the group homes again, but didn't want to rush into making a quick decision. "I will know it when I see it," I said. I kept praying for an answer, trying to find messages in the readings and homilies at church. I tried to connect with my mother in the heavens above and ask her for her help. I knew how much she adored Lee, so I knew she would always be his guardian angel. Sometimes it brought me to tears, but I kept at it, looking for special messages from other people who also dealt with this quandary. I wasn't the first person who had to find a home for a son ... *Why was this so difficult?*

I visited a group home on the sly without telling my family. I wanted to process, without their input, the whole picture of what it would be like for Lee to live away from the only home he has ever known. The boys were very disappointed in my decision to visit homes without them, and felt somewhat betrayed that I didn't invite them to join me. So, I agreed to have them accompany me in the future.

I revisited the Life Sharing experience with Felix and his wife, Kathy. Felix was Lee's companion, and Lee was quite comfortable being around both Felix and Kathy. They were already Life Sharing with another individual, and I thought that person might provide companionship for Lee. After we started the preliminary paperwork, however, Felix called to tell me he had a family emergency and would not be able to provide for Lee. I told him not to worry, that it wasn't meant to be. Looking back, I feel that this divine intervention allowed me to keep looking for the right placement for Lee.

My phone call to Lee's social worker the following day to tell him about our fallen plans came with a big surprise. The social worker informed me that a person representing Dayspring Homes called him to say he was very interested in having Lee come to live at one of their houses. *What? Did I hear him correctly?* I always knew that if Dayspring Homes ever became available, I would certainly consider that for Lee.

Dayspring Homes was started by a Catholic nun who realized the dilemma of so many aging parents. What do parents do with their grown children when they are no longer able to care for those children? She realized the sacrifices these parents have made over the years to care for their disabled children, so she started a group home to provide services for several individuals.

I was aware of the Dayspring Homes and tried many times to visit to see if it might be a good fit for Lee, but I was always told the waiting list was so incredibly long that it would not be worthwhile to pursue it. What I didn't know was that Dayspring Homes had grown from one home to five homes. There was an opening at one of those five homes, and the administrators wanted to meet my son. I immediately let the social worker know that I was definitely interested in going to visit the house. *Could my prayers be answered?*

Lee, John, Matt, Billy, and I met at the group home on a Friday afternoon on a cold winter day, exactly two years since my first encounter with the group home concept. I wasn't sure what to expect, but I knew what I wanted to see.

It was located in the town where I grew up, and I kept praying as we drove to Shillington. I really couldn't believe that for so long I had wondered what to do for him, and now we were possibly going to find out.

We were greeted by the friendly house staff, the Dayspring supervisor, the social worker, and three lovely residents. They were all so friendly and welcoming. There were pictures of the residents on the walls and carpeting on the floors! There was a feeling of welcome wherever I looked. It felt good. We were given a tour of the modest rancher and then taken to the downstairs to what could be Lee's living quarters. We were shown a bedroom, a bathroom, and a very spacious living room. All of this space could be Lee's. It could be his bachelor pad!

It was a very quiet environment, as the other residents had similar requests for calm. They enjoyed gatherings, but preferred the peace and solitude of their own intimate spaces. We discussed various opportunities that Lee could be afforded if he came to live there. They would continue his trips to the gym, take him to his weekly swimming lessons, visit local malls, and find time to bowl and have parties. It really was exactly what I had been requesting in prayer for all these years!

After our visit, we went for dinner and drinks to discuss the possibility of Lee's new home. We all were amazed at the opportunity this presented for Lee, and none of us saw anything we didn't like about the home. We agreed as a family that Lee would live there if all the paperwork was approved.

Many tears fell when Lee was accepted to this Dayspring Home. Lee would soon be moving out of the only home he had ever known for almost forty-four years. This new home truly was the answer to all my prayers, and I have come to realize—as I had always been taught—that God listens to prayers and answers them in his time. Sometimes the answers are not what we asked for or what we hoped for, but they are nevertheless answered. After much conversation with my wonderful guys, I was at peace with our decision.

In order to make the transition as easy as possible for Lee, we started by taking baby steps. Lee and I were first invited to a wonderful spaghetti dinner at the home. All of the residents attended. As in the Catholic tradition, the group said grace, beginning with the sign of the cross. I could see that it was a tradition that occurred before their evening meals, and I was comforted by this expression of faith. I was pleased with the easy flow of meaningful conversation, and Lee was totally at ease with both the residents and the staff. He eventually left the table to sit nearby and watch TV. After dinner, we thanked everyone for a wonderful evening and left the house with a feeling of gratitude and with no anxiety. Matt and Billy called the following morning and were both surprised that I was at peace with the previous night's experience.

We followed up our dinner with an overnight visit. The bedroom had a bed in it for respite services, so we planned for a Friday night stay. Lee questioned what was happening, but didn't seem fearful or anxious. He took some of his favorite things with him: his alarm clock, his calculator, and his favorite tapes for his old tape recorder. That night John and I had a relaxing evening and I waited through the night until I could see Lee the next day and observe his body language. All seemed well with absolutely no visible evidence that he struggled with the change.

Our next step was a weekend visit. We chose an elongated visit on Presidents' Day weekend in February. Coincidentally, it was the same weekend that John and the guys had planned to go to the mountains, which meant I would be alone in our house. Lee always hung out with me when the guys went away, so I wanted to keep busy and try not to dwell on thoughts of Lee.

My daughter-in-law invited me to dinner and a movie on Friday evening, and I jumped at the chance for a diversion. On Saturday I devoted my time to projects for Lee's new living quarters: painting a mirror purchased at a thrift store, framing family pictures for his walls, sewing curtains for his windows, and finishing the final stitches of a patchwork quilt for his bed. Working into the wee hours of the morning and keeping busy allowed me to stay positive and process my thoughts through work. I had the mindset that Lee was going away to college just as his brothers had done many years before. I was getting his dorm ready!

When I picked up Lee after the long weekend, I realized that he was fine. I'd like to think that he missed me a bit, but then again I hoped he didn't and that he would realize that there is so much more to life than living with his parents! He enjoyed his time with the others, and the staff assured me that he adjusted beautifully.

Knowing that this was truly what Lee wanted, I was able to come to terms with my own feelings of sadness and loneliness so long as Lee was happy. It was difficult for me to comprehend not having that aspect of my life anymore after taking care of Lee for so many years. I knew that letting him go was going to be a tremendous adjustment for me.

The following Monday, after talking to the social worker, the date was set. Saturday, March 25, was Lee's move-in day. I started shopping for new sheets for his bed, new towels for his bathroom, a shower curtain, and rugs for the floor. The living room of Lee's new space was a dark brown paneling, so I decided to paint it before his move. I needed three full days to complete the project, but it also gave me a good feeling knowing that I was sprucing up his home. I felt as though I was leaving a part of me in his new dwelling place. I wanted his new environment to be as comfortable as possible.

While I worked I was comforted by the quiet chatter of the staff, as I could hear them enjoying their work. The residents were at their day program and their caregivers were doing the laundry, paperwork, and light cleaning. It was a snowy morning and, as I looked out the window of his home that was nestled on the edge of the woods, I felt calmness for Lee. The deer came within feet of the home and squirrels and birds frolicked about. It was so peaceful. I envisioned the furnishings for his space and really couldn't wait for his move, as I knew it was time.

After so much planning, Lee's moving day was finally upon us. It was a sunny morning and I made a special breakfast for the guys as we started the process. Lee kept asking me as he struggled with some of the boxes, "Mom, what are we doing?" I replied with a smile and tears. "Lee, you are moving to Hillside!" "Yes Mom," he replied. He was reaffirming to me that he was okay with this.

Our caravan included two pick-up trucks and our car filled to the brim with Lee's belongings. Throughout the previous week, I had already taken a lot of his clothes and incidentals over to the house, so that we mostly had to worry about the big items for the main move. The curtains were hung, the bed was in place, and new bedding adorned it. I felt proud for him to have such a beautiful living area. We finished our project by lunchtime.

As we finished hanging the last pictures on the walls, Lee was invited to go bowling with the residents. When he was asked to join them, he hesitated and looked at me for reassurance. I assured him that he should go and have fun and that I would see him soon. It really was perfect timing. The staff helped me say good-bye to him in the best possible way. I gave him a big hug as he left on his way to start his new life. It wasn't easy, and I felt the mother's heartache of watching my child set out on his own. But I was thrilled that Lee was on his way to finding the fulfilling life I always hoped for him.

I waited a week until I went to see Lee for the first time, since I didn't want him to think I was coming to take him home if I came for him midweek. Billy and his two young sons went with me to pick Lee up to take him to our grandson's birthday party. I couldn't wait to see him. When he opened the door, I was taken aback. Lee had a mustache! *What on earth!* "Oh Lee, what is that?" I questioned. "Yes Mom," was his reply once again. Lee was learning independence!

My days are very different without Lee. I think of him throughout the day and wonder if he might at some time think of me too. My family couldn't be happier with our choice for his placement, and after a few hours running around town with me on the weekend, he is quite happy to head home to his own pad. There will be trials for him and for us in the years to come, but he is surrounded with compassionate people who will care for his needs almost as well as his mother did.

Most moms experience the feeling of separation from their children, some sooner and some later. I just hoped that Lee understood everything we were doing for him was for his happiness in life.

CHAPTER 16:
CONTRIBUTING TO SOCIETY

When Lee lost his position at Boscov's and we were unsuccessful in finding him employment elsewhere, we reluctantly decided to pursue employment for Lee at Prospectus Berco, a sheltered workshop. Sheltered workshops, now referred to as work centers, employ people with disabilities at sub-minimum wages and provide a place for people with limited intellect to work and contribute to society. Quite frankly, I always had higher expectations for Lee and struggled to accept that he wasn't able to re-enter the real world of work. He had been successful at Boscov's for so many years with the help and support of compassionate co-workers, and I hoped and prayed that the pieces of the puzzle would again fit together for things to fall into place for Lee.

As the years passed, Lee continued the day-to-day grind of working on sporadic tasks at the sheltered workshop, sometimes earning a take-home pay of $2 every two weeks. Losing hope that he'd ever again be gainfully employed, I assumed this was what he would do until his retirement.

Lee had so much to offer; there had to be a job for him that was geared to his strength of repetition, repetition, repetition, a job that most people would not like to do. Though he was not able to multitask, I was sure he could work all day long and thrive if working alone on a specific task because he sees a task that he does over and over the same as if he only started it for the first time. But time went by, and those chances of Lee finding his perfect job seemed to be fading away. It was as though "his ship had sailed," which is what someone said to me one day.

After Lee moved into his group home and settled into his new surroundings and family, I was approached about a new concept for hard-to-place disabled people who were looking for employment. The Goodwill Employment Agency had started a new program that incorporated customized employment. Referred to as the Discovery Program, it was directed to employers open to the concept of hiring an individual for a specific task, not someone who would have to multitask. It sounded interesting, but I did not allow myself to get too excited about it.

Once again, Lee was in the job market. We proceeded with the concept cautiously, measuring Lee's strengths once again. Through the years, I had updated Lee's resume, filled out job applications for him, and talked to prospective employers. Thankfully, in later years Matt and Billy helped me with these tasks. With an abundance of computer and communication skills, they were able to clearly articulate to potential employers Lee's strengths and shortcomings.

Months went by, and I actually forgot about the Discovery Program. Then one day I received a phone call from Lee's social worker, who told me there might be an opportunity for him. I showed appreciation to the social worker, but assumed it would fall through yet again.

This opportunity, however, was different. A possible employer had been found. A family-owned company had a position for someone who'd be willing to bag three small batteries in a plastic bag. They actually hired Lee because of his work experience.

Lee now gets up four days a week, takes a taxi cab to his place of employment, and successfully completes his required tasks for his employer. In addition to bagging batteries, he also builds small circuit boards, which are used in manufacturing flashlights. He initially had a job coach to ease him into his new environment and required tasks, but Lee has been so successful in this position that his job coach only checks in with him occasionally to make sure all is well.

Lee has the support of his co-workers and his employer if any small problems arise, and their encouragement is vital in order for him to achieve his goals. This job has been the culmination of Lee's lifetime search for the perfect job for his abilities. He's an absolute success!

We have come full circle. After forty-eight years of hoping for the best for our son, our mission has been accomplished. He is a contributing member of society as a working man, and feeling very good about himself. Our family is so very proud of his accomplishments.

CHAPTER 17:

REFLECTION AND HOPE

When Lee was first diagnosed in 1976, autism was just being mentioned and explored by doctors. Oddly, looking back, I honestly wonder if our early doctors knew anything at all about it. I am struck with the quick and curt advice they gave with little to no knowledge or familiarity with the affliction. I am glad I only took their advice in select and measured doses when it felt right in my soul.

There were parents who actually did send their children to institutions, like we were told to do with Lee. These children seemed to have more severe symptoms than Lee presented. Some smeared their feces on the walls at night while their families were sleeping; others hurt themselves by banging their heads against the walls. Though I never did and never will judge other parents because of their choices, I could not fathom the idea of not being a part of my child's day-to-day living.

Thankfully, Lee did not do any harm to his body. In fact, because he was overly cautious, he has never had a real scrape or bruise on his legs or arms. He was not destructive in the home. He just seemed to enjoy life in his own little world, and I was committed to making that world be all it could be for him. I am amazed at how far Lee has come since it was recommended that he should go to an institution.

The possibilities of great improvement for children who are now given an autistic diagnosis are endless. The interventions and therapies that they receive will be the key to their improvements. If you are the parent of a child with a disability, reach out and get help as soon as you realize there is something that is not quite right in your child's behavior. You will always have to be your child's voice, their advocate. There will be plenty of professionals who will say "no" to you, but you must be the one to say "yes" for your child.

There will always be people who do not get it. They have no idea what people with disabilities are dealing with on a daily basis. Their minds might be closed to the disenfranchised. It is our calling to be the example, to show them.

Quite honestly, it took me a long time to come to grips with autism and Lee. It is difficult to deal with what you do not understand. It took me so very long to comprehend exactly how Lee was feeling and the challenges he was trying to overcome. When I tried something new for Lee, I always thought this would be it, the cure, but over and over again, I was disappointed.

Looking back over my more than seventy years, I know that God has always had His plan for me, my purpose in life. It has taken me my lifetime to understand His intentions. We are formed by life's situations, whether for the good or for the bad. How we use our God-given skills and abilities will determine how we deal with challenges in life's journey. For me, I see a few formative areas that allowed me to help Lee the best I could.

- My amazing childhood of warmth, love, and happiness formed my basic personality. It enabled me to see the positive much more than the negative.

- The desire to compete that I developed through participating in athletics as a child and throughout my life enabled me to keep digging into difficult situations instead of surrendering to them.

- My belief in God and my constant prayers gave me an inner strength and belief that everything would be okay. My mother's constant reminder to "say your prayers" formed who I am and what I believe.

- The chance of meeting a man who had solid family roots and an unbelievable stubbornness in his DNA to not give up reinforced my commitment to meeting challenges. His undying love for family and his ability to keep his head up energized me and gave me the fuel I needed to keep moving onward.

I thank God every day for the blessings he has given me: John Henry, Matthew John, Lee Jonathan, William David, Kelly Sue, Kelly Elizabeth, Zachary Brian, Benjamin Matthew, Abigail Mary, Brady John, and Colin William. They all played an enormous part in Lee's outcome. Words cannot express the amount of love I have in my heart for all of them. It was our whole family that helped Lee to overcome his challenges to succeed.

What is my advice to young mothers who might experience their child's diagnosis of autism?

- Reach out. You are not alone. There are so many advocacy groups eager to help you.
- Reach in. Find that inner strength that you probably don't recognize yet. It's there. You must find it. You are your child's voice.
- Stay committed. You will have disappointments and setbacks but keep looking ahead.
- Take time for yourself. Find what relaxes you and do it. Stay with it!
- Try to laugh to keep from crying, but know it is ok to cry.
- Make each of your children feel special. It is not always easy to find time, but please take the time. You will be repaid a thousand fold in years to come.
- Trust in God. Whatever spiritual belief you have, take time to nurture it. Daily prayer or reflections will help you deal with what is going to be a very long and unbelievably interesting road that you will travel!
- Embrace it! It is a wonderful world!

Challenges that I never knew existed until Lee, helped me appreciate the challenges of others who were dealing with much more than what I have had to deal with in my life. Be the difference in your corner of the world. Be the difference in someone else's life. As Pope Francis said, "To change the world we must be good to those who cannot repay us."

Motherhood doesn't stop when a child enters a certain age. It is a forever, innate feeling. I will forever have Lee on my mind. I still remind him not to stare at pretty girls and not to act inappropriately. But now it's not because I don't want him to embarrass me, it's because I don't want him to embarrass himself. I have always said, "It is not easy being Lee, but he is amazing at it!!"

AFTERWORD

As the years have gone by, I realize that Lee will always see new experiences as stressful events, but they will be manageable. Routine situations will always feel like new experiences for him. He will always see things exactly as they are; he will not understand abstract thinking. He will never be rushed, but will instead go through life with only one speed—low gear.

Giving up daily caregiving to someone else doesn't mean that I gave up all aspects of Lee's life. I am still his advocate whenever I see he needs one. I still keep my ear to the ground to find new opportunities or benefits that will help him in his future. As long as I live and breathe, I will have Lee's best interest in my heart and mind.

To me, family is everything. When I look at the men that Matt and Billy have become, I could not be more proud. These two boys have gone through life learning alongside me. They acquired skills in coping with difficult situations, as well as difficult people. Their compassion for those less fortunate and those who are marginalized is admirable.

The love and care they showed to their brother throughout the years are reflected in the love and care they show to their own families. They know the right thing to do when raising their children and loving their wives. It is often said that men treat their wives the way they treat their mothers. I am so blessed to have been their mother. I thank God every day for His guidance in raising my boys.

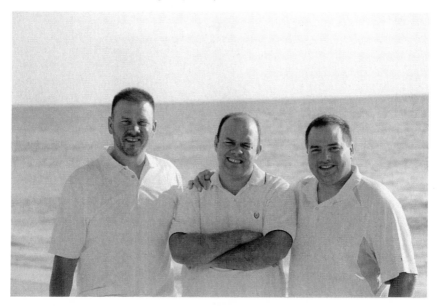

"The Ruth Boys"

John and I watch from a distance how secure they are in their positions as husbands, fathers, and businessmen. The enjoyment they receive from their children reminds me of the circle of life and how they are continuing what we started for them. I know with certainty that Lee will be fine because Matt and Billy will always look after him. Wherever he goes, whatever evolves in his living situation and in his life, he will have two very caring brothers overseeing his happiness. *God Bless You.*

When Billy's daughter thanked me one day for "raising such a cool dad," it made me realize how much her Uncle

Lee had an influence in that outcome. With awe, I look at what all our family has learned from this incredible ride with this amazing man.

Thirty-five years later, that vibrator is still in our attic! I better clean out the attic before someone other than my husband or sons comes across that therapy basket!

ACKNOWLEDGEMENTS

There have been so many people who have influenced me and encouraged me over the forty-plus years of my journey as Lee's mother. While not possible to mention all of the wonderful points of light, I would like to thank those who were key and instrumental in making this book a reality.

- Thank you, Beryll, for planting the seed.
- Thank you, Lori, for getting my story cultivated.
- Thank you, Matt, for all of your weeding and thinning.
- Thank you, Kelly E. and Nancy, for your amazing ability to pick and sort the product.

I am forever grateful.

Linda / Mom / Aunt

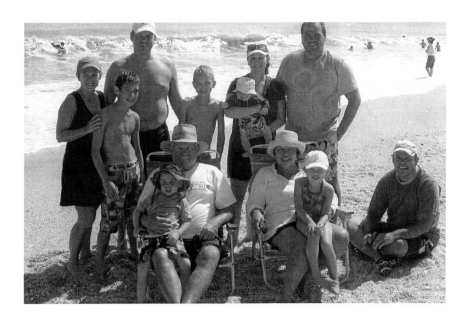

"The Ruth Family in Cape May"